WHAT PEOPLE ARE SAYING ABOUT

SWEETENING THE PILL

Holly Grigg-Spall is fearless, and her courageous advocacy on behalf of women whose stories are too often silenced is a model for others trying to make positive change through health activism. Read the book and get inspired, get angry, and most importantly get information. *Sweetening the Pill* is exactly the thing needed to energize and mobilize this important women's health conversation.

Laura Eldridge, author of *In Our Control: The Complete Guide to Contraceptive Choices for Women*, co-author and co-editor with Barbara Seaman of *The No-Nonsense Guide to Menopause* and co-editor, again with Barbara Seaman, of *Voices of the Women's Health Movement*.

In *Sweetening the Pill* Holly Grigg-Spall lays out the reality of hormonal contraception, and the ubiquitous political and commercial interests at play, with breathtaking precision. With most young women using these drugs, and providers cynically side-stepping informed consent and respectful consultation, this is a core and urgent issue of our time. If you are interested in teen girl and womens' health, and the wellbeing and evolution of society as a whole read *Sweetening the Pill*. It's a riveting read and a powerful tool for change.

Jane Bennett, co-author of *The Pill: Are You Sure It's For You?*, *The Natural Fertility Management Contraception Kit* and *A Blessing Not A Curse*.

Holly Grigg-Spall effectively melts the candy coating that obscures a simple truth: what we don't know, can indeed hurt us. *Sweetening the Pill*, equal parts personal journey, investigative journalism and feminist manifesto, cracks open the paternalist and corporate-driven ethos of self-improvement that undermines women's body literacy. We've got to demand better: more transparency, more options and more support for self-determined health care. Getting there begins with the kind of courageous inquiry Grigg-Spall inspires.

Chris Bobel, associate professor of Women's Studies at University of Massachusetts Boston and author of *New Blood: Third Wave Feminism and the Politics of Menstruation* and *The Paradox of Natural Mothering*.

We discovered in the '70s that the personal is political. Holly Grigg-Spall starts with her and other women's personal experiences with the pill, then thoughtfully and thoroughly considers it scientifically, medically and philosophically to discover the political truth of the pill. She shares strategies for finding new ways to control our fertility while regaining control of our destiny. Grigg-Spall's careful study on the pill's effect on women's health is long, long overdue. We are so busy fighting to keep hormonal birth control available that we don't want to question what it is doing to our health and our lives. After reading this book, we can never see the pill in the same way again.

Carol Downer, is a veteran women's health activist and author of *A New View of a Woman's Body, How to Stay Out of the Gynecologist's Office, A Woman's Book of Choices* and *Woman Centered Pregnancy and Birth*. She serves on the Board of Directors of the Feminist Women's Health Centers of California, which operates eight Women's Health Specialists clinics.

Oral contraceptives have done so much for so many, but when they don't stand up to scrutiny, women have a right to know more. *Sweetening The Pill* is a fascinating and up-to-the-minute account of the persistent questions around the effects of birth control pills. Holly Grigg-Spall's cross-cultural perspective provides keen insights into the impact of the latest US health care initiatives. Consolidating personal testimonies, current thought and the controversy surrounding the widespread and prolonged use of oral contraception, this book is a toolkit for action.

Chella Quint, is a writer, educator and performer at Adventures in Menstruating.

Sweetening the Pill

or How We Got Hooked on Hormonal Birth Control

Sweetening the Pill

or How We Got Hooked on Hormonal Birth Control

Holly Grigg-Spall

zero
books

Winchester, UK
Washington, USA

First published by Zero Books, 2013
Zero Books is an imprint of John Hunt Publishing Ltd., Laurel House, Station Approach,
Alresford, Hants, SO24 9JH, UK
office1@jhpbooks.net
www.johnhuntpublishing.com
www.zero-books.net

For distributor details and how to order please visit the 'Ordering' section on our website.

Text copyright: Holly Grigg-Spall 2013

ISBN: 978 1 78099 607 3

A CIP catalogue record for this book is available from the British Library.

Design: Stuart Davies

Printed in the USA by Edwards Brothers Malloy

We operate a distinctive and ethical publishing philosophy in all
areas of our business, from our global network of authors to
production and worldwide distribution.

CONTENTS

Dedication

For every woman who has suffered physically and emotionally as a result of hormonal birth control.

Acknowledgments

I am going to thank just a few of those who have given me encouragement and support, although there have certainly been many more who have given their time, conversation and guidance and so contributed to this book. Thanks to Laura Wershler for her collaboration and determination; Elizabeth Kissling for welcoming me into the Society for Menstrual Cycle Research and providing the fantastic re:Cycling blog; Geraldine Matus for her edits and suggestions; Alexandra Pope and Jane Bennett for the book that first opened my eyes; Laura Eldridge for tracking me down; editor at The Independent Louisa Saunders for believing in what I had to say along with Jessica Stites at Ms. and the health editors at Easy Living; all those who wrote angry comments on my Bitch blog posts and so trained me to defend my position; Mt Holyoke college for planting a seed in my mind; Laura Tricker for sharing her story; my mum and dad for their backing; Molly Butterworth for her time and thoughts; Laura Holness for figuring things out with me in that Asda parking lot years ago, and all of the women who've contributed to my blog, told me their stories and thanked me for speaking out. Thank you to my husband Guy for encouraging me to just write and not wait to be asked, for supporting me in my decision, and for sticking with me through the worst of it.

Foreword

In a letter dated March 22, 1980, I proposed to the editor of an American woman's magazine that they consider my enclosed article: The Contraceptive Dilemma - A Subjective Appraisal of the Status of Birth Control.

I wrote: "Recent articles (about birth control) deal almost exclusively with the basic pros, cons, and how-tos of the various contraceptives available - matter-of-fact discussions that reduce birth control to a mere pragmatic decision. If only that were the case. Contraception, like the sexual interaction that necessitates it, involves our emotions as much as it does the facts. Yet the subjective, personal aspect of contraception is so often ignored. In this age of scientific research we are expected to (subjugate) our emotional reactions to significant probabilities, our anger to logic. Very real fears and earnest questions are dismissed as irrelevant...."

Although today I wouldn't use the phrase "emotional reactions," it's hard to believe that three decades later, the status of birth control and women's relationship to it has not much changed. Websites, not magazines, now host information about the basic pros, cons and how-tos of available birth control methods. But it is writers like Holly, half my age, who honor women's real fears and ask earnest questions that are still being dismissed as mostly irrelevant.

Just as my personal story with the pill - including over a year of distressing post-pill amenorrhea - set me on a course of research and advocacy, so too has Holly's personal experience. *Sweetening the Pill* explores and challenges the ways in which the pill and other drug-based contraceptives damage women's health, threaten our autonomy and thwart body literacy. What we don't know about our bodies helps pharmaceutical companies "sell" their contraceptive drugs, and keeps us "addicted" to them.

At some point between my first attempt at non-hormonal contraceptive advocacy and Holly's exploration of how we've become hooked on hormonal birth control, something disturbing transpired. Prescribing the pill, or other forms of hormonal contraception, has become, in the minds of most health-care providers, the "standard of care" for being a girl. It is all too common to subjugate a girl's menstrual cycle to synthetic hormones that superficially "regulate," but actually suspend the maturation of her reproductive system. And for many girls, the use of hormonal contraception continues well into their 20s, without awareness of what might be or has been sacrificed.

There are many women like Holly who are fed up with hormonal birth control. I've met scores of them during my 30 years involvement within the mainstream pro-choice sexual and reproductive health community, the one that prides itself on inclusion and diversity. Yet I've been unsuccessful in my constant advocacy for this community to accommodate a more inclusive, diverse approach to contraception, to provide acknowledgment, support and services to women who can't, won't or don't want to use hormonal contraceptive methods. We pay lip service to the idea, but the message we convey is: "You're on your own."

I've found enthusiasm in other realms for my menstrual cycle advocacy and my belief that many women want to, and can, learn to use non-hormonal methods effectively and confidently. I've found scientific evidence of the value of ovulation to women's health and well-being.

I've read, met or worked with several of the sources included in this book. Many have devoted their careers to understanding women's bodies and our relationships with our bodies in ways the medical mainstream typically ignores and barely comprehends. They have made contributions that help us imagine a different way of thinking about fertility, contraception and our menstrual cycles in relation to our sexual, reproductive and overall health.

I like to think that all of our work provides the framework, reason and evidence to support Holly's decision and the decision of hundreds of thousands of women who want to or have already said "No" to hormonal birth control.

Sweetening the Pill is an important book because it speaks to young women who intuitively, subconsciously, or actively are leaning in this direction. It offers a contemporary perspective on the pill and its influence on our bodies and our lives, as well as evidence that affirms and confirms the sacrifices we make - large and small - to live under its influence. It remains for readers to decide what to do about it.

Laura Wershler

Laura Wershler writes, speaks and advocates on a broad range of sexual and reproductive health issues. She currently writes a weekly women's health column for Troymedia.com. Follow her on Twitter @laurawershler.

Contact
hollygriggspall@gmail.com
@hollygriggspall
www.sweeteningthepill.com
original blog: www.sweeteningthepill.blogspot.com

Introduction: It's Not Me

When I returned to the doctor who had prescribed me the birth control pill Yasmin three years earlier I told her that I had spent the time since slowly unraveling. I had whirled through many levels of misery before realizing that my choice of contraception could be the cause. Yasmin was the third oral contraceptive I had taken in a decade. I was seventeen when I popped the first pill.

The doctor listened quietly and then said, "I took the pill for twenty years. When I came off it, I realized I was a completely different person to who I'd thought. I had been depressed the whole time and now I'm much, much happier."

She then suggested I give a different brand, Femodette, a try. Although puzzled, I conceded and took her prescription.

Yasmin was released in 2001 by the pharmaceutical company Bayer Pharmaceuticals and followed by its descendent Yaz in 2006. They are different from other pill brands because they contain a new progestin (synthetic progesterone) component, drospirenone. I started taking Yasmin in 2006 when it seemed as though every woman I knew was doing the same.

After graduating from college in the UK I spent some months in San Francisco where I saw the television commercials that pronounced this new birth control pill as capable of combating everything from PMS to bloating to acne. Currently there are a number of drospirenone-containing pills available, including generics – Beyaz, Yasminelle, Ocella, Zarah, Angeliq, Syeda, Safyral, Gianvi and Loryna.

The marketing hype filtered from the US through to the UK, where I was presented with this popular new drug by my GP when the pill I had been taking started to make me bleed badly during sex. The women's magazines that I read hinted at Yasmin's skin-clearing, weight-loss and breast-enhancing effects. My doctor said Yasmin was the very latest model, modernized and therefore superior to all other brands. Word of mouth spread about this wonder drug and it became a must-have. Women I knew gushed about their perfect skin and their need for bigger bras. They said they had lost ten pounds. Both my sisters and my best friend were taking it along with many other friends and colleagues. This was the first time I had heard women discuss a type of pill by name.

Previously the brand names for pills only came into conversation because of negative controversy. I had heard that Dianette, although prescribed for acne, caused depression and blood clots. In a short time Yasmin, and then Yaz, became the most popular pills worldwide despite being the most expensive on the market. It was a diet drug, a beauty product and a contraceptive all rolled into one, and doctor endorsed to boot.

I was two years into taking Yasmin when a friend confessed to me that she had been feeling very down. She said she felt like her head was filled with cotton wool. She felt detached from life, her interest in sex had disappeared, and so had her interest in everything else she had previously enjoyed. When I heard this I admitted that I too had been feeling depressed for some time. I felt my confidence and energy was evaporating. I had little motivation and struggled to think clearly. I had stopped reading and found it harder and harder to write, which was impacting on my work.

We agreed that our skin had never looked better, we were the thinnest we'd ever been and we'd long left behind our B cups, but we were both really unhappy. My friend brought up Dianette, recalling the reports that it caused depression.

"Do you think this could all be because of Yasmin?" she asked.

I did not disclose the full extent of my unhappiness. I did not tell her about the bouts of anxiety and paranoia that had me at home alone calling my boyfriend twice an hour to check he wasn't dead and caused me to leave parties convinced I had burned all bridges with my friends. Nor did I mention the constant sense of dread that convinced me that some terrible event was always just around the corner and had me visualizing disasters and tragedies. I didn't talk about the spasms of rage that led to fights that lasted for hours and stopped only in exhaustion. These swings of extreme emotion had insidiously spread from occupying a week per month to every day of my life. I had weekly breakdowns when I would spiral into deep, hopeless depression, racked with insecurities and unfathomable anger to the point that I'd become completely unmoored from reality and unable to see a way out of my thinking.

I didn't tell her that I thought I was losing my mind.

After that conversation I began researching and found out that Yasmin and Yaz were amongst the most complained about drugs on the Internet. Women in online forums described experiences that were eerily similar to my own. Their minds hooked on to the same anxieties and they reacted with the same heightened emotions, which scared and confused them. They described experiencing a complete change in personality. They distrusted their partners, friends and families. Panic attacks became so frequent they were in a constant state of fear. Chronic fatigue kept them from leaving the house and for some lost them their job or their relationship. I found a forum specifically for users of my birth control called the Yaz Survivors Forum.

In the US Yasmin and Yaz were promoted as what *The New York Times* dubbed "a quality of life treatment" and this message was enthusiastically taken up in the UK by doctors, family planning clinics and women themselves. The two pills differ only in the length of their monthly break. Yaz was promoted specifically as a treatment for the anxiety and depression associated with PMS and the controversial newly created disorder Premenstrual Dysphoric Disorder (PMDD) – defined as a more serious form of PMS. These drugs prevented pregnancy at the same rate as all other oral contraceptives and so were made to stand out via an aggressive marketing campaign.

After a year of Bayer's hyperbolic claims circulating, the FDA requested that the company distribute a corrective television advertisement. Bayer, they ruled, had made misleading assertions about the capabilities of these highly profitable drugs. Yaz was openly promoted for unapproved uses and the television commercials made light of the serious health risks like blood clots. These pills had the potential to produce a life-threatening level of potassium in the blood, a unique facet that Bayer had declined to make clear publicly.

Yet the company's guarded retraction did little to impact the sales. In 2010 Bayer made $1.5 billion from Yaz, then its second best-selling product.

As I researched I wondered exactly how these drugs achieved their most alluring effects. I wondered precisely how the skin clearing, weight-loss and breasts-enhancement were engineered in my body. I had never considered that the pill could have a whole body effect, but the changes were too obvious to ignore. There was something about what these pills provided that women wanted and needed that kept them asking for and taking them. We were convinced by the external signs of apparent good health. I thought that looking good equaled feeling good and being healthy.

I didn't stop taking Yasmin right then. Instead I pitched a feature article to *Easy Living* magazine entitled 'What You Should Know About The Pill' that was based on an interview with Dr Cynthia Graham, a research scientist affiliated with the Kinsey Institute. I had only written film and culture journalism previously but felt the need to get this information, any information out.

I could not understand how I had never read anything about the pill's emotional side effects. A Kinsey Institute study found that half of all women experienced negative mood changes on the pill. Dr Graham told me that, in her opinion, the pervasiveness of the pill was founded on a "gender bias" within the medical industry. She said this in a manner so matter-of-fact that it was not until I saw the quote printed in the magazine that I was struck by its seriousness.

Writing this piece was a struggle. I was still taking Yasmin and my brain fog, lack of concentration and fatigue combined to make the process like wading through mud. I was finding it near impossible to convert my fuzzy thinking into a clear, relatively simple article.

My experience taking Yasmin drew my attention to hormonal contraceptives as a whole. I had not until that point considered exactly why I took the pill since I had always asked my partners to use condoms. I spent so long blaming myself for my breakdowns, not considering they could be down to the drug I was taking every day. I was forced to confront my feelings about the pill and as a part of that to look at my relationship to my body.

After the article was published, I swapped to Femodette for three months and then came off the pill completely for two months.

As well as my disintegrating mental health, I noted the numerous physical problems I suffered – regular urinary tract infections, sore and bleeding gums, hypoglycemic symptoms, hair loss, and muscle weakness to name just some. I began to consider that these problems might also be rooted in my long-term birth control pill use. I had learnt more about the pill in one summer than I had known in the many years prior.

In the few months I took off the pill I felt lighter. A rush of positive emotions let me feel happiness, excitement and enthusiasm. I became stable in both my thoughts and feelings. I felt stronger, more confident and far less fearful. I reconnected with the world. I had clarity of thinking that allowed me to engage again. On the pill I felt stagnant and still, when I was not in the throes of breakdown. In the times of respite, I was tired and deadened.

Yet, like a victim of Stockholm Syndrome I returned to taking it.

I popped the pill again one morning because it felt like the right thing to do. I rationalized my decision even though the change in me had been so obvious. Taking the pill every morning was all I had known for so long and not doing it made me uneasy. I worried that not taking the pill would change my relationship and leave me in a constant state of anxiety over whether or not I was pregnant. The mental turmoil I had gone through on Yasmin left me unable to think well for myself. I did not have the strength of mind or character at that time to go against years of indoctrination.

I moved to the US with my American boyfriend and we got married. There I started a blog. Within a few weeks of chronicling Yasmin's impact on my mood and well-being in the hope of helping others, I began to receive comments and emails from women who had also suffered from these side effects. I heard from someone I had known back in school and she described her own experience coming off the pill after ten years as "life changing."

I started reading the book *The Pill: Are You Sure It's For You?* By Jane Bennett and Alexandra Pope and it was this paragraph that shook me awake: "By altering our natural hormone levels, the pill induces in us a *different* biochemical and psychological state. This in turn interferes with the particular psychological stage of life we're in and may affect our unfoldment thereafter…While it may be difficult to prove the effect that taking the pill has on our psychological development we can see that through its profound hormonal impact the pill may also be interfering with the fundamental chemistry of who we are and what we can become."

It was then that I decided to stop taking the pill for good.

In the blog I would detail how this transition unfolded. After ten years I stopped with no idea of how this might affect me. I logged every detail of this transformative and tumultuous time. As my mind cleared and my energy returned I eagerly delved deeper into the world of hormonal contraceptives.

Two years later, in 2011, the FDA entered into a reappraisal of Bayer's and all drospirenone-containing oral contraceptives. Five research studies were released that showed these drugs hold a fifty to seventy-five percent increased risk of causing blood clots in comparison with pills containing other progestins. Two studies released by Bayer in the years prior had claimed the drugs held no higher risk than other birth control pills on the market.

A former FDA commissioner, David Kessler, charged that Bayer deliberately withheld data about the blood clot risk rates early on in the FDA approval process in order to push the drugs quickly onto the market. He claimed that Bayer had used underhand marketing techniques to convince women that Yaz and Yasmin were cure-all drugs, fuelling their popularity. He accused Bayer of paying women's magazines to advocate for the pills and pay rolling experts to promote them in their books and talks. Aware that only through striking differentiation could these pills become more profitable than others Bayer had pulled women in with the superficial benefits without declaring the extent of the potential pay-off.

The FDA called an advisory committee to evaluate the safety of these pills, which included the generic versions created since Bayer's patent expired. The decision of the committee had the potential to cause these drugs to be pulled off the market completely. However, the panel voted by a four-person margin that the drugs' benefits outweighed the risks.

A government watchdog group, the Project on Government Oversight conducted an independent investigation that revealed three of the advisors on the FDA panel had financial ties to Bayer. A fourth advisor was connected financially to the manufacturing of the generic versions. All four voted for Yaz, Yasmin and all other drospirenone-containing pills to continue to be prescribed by doctors without restriction. POGO requested that the FDA assemble a new advisory committee with no conflicts of interest to make another assessment.

The FDA did not respond to this request, instead it was decided that a statement be added to the insert declaring the discovery of "conflicting" research that suggested the pills might hold a higher risk of causing blood clots. The statement acknowledged the conclusions of the research funded by Bayer and gives it equal standing to the contrasting research performed by other bodies, including the FDA itself. Providing this warning has the intention of protecting doctors and the pharmaceutical companies from responsibility for the safety of the drugs' users.

As this process was underway, for the first known time in US history, a Republican candidate in the running for Presidency – Rick Santorum – voiced support for a state-led ban on the use of birth control. The call for health insurance companies and employers to provide contraception through President Obama's Affordable Care Act had ignited a frenzied debate over access to birth control that was powered by anti-abortion groups and the religious Right.

The FDA investigation and decision over drospirenone-containing pills was barely reported in the media. In contrast, the threat to access provoked women to type tirades and take to the streets. The terms 'birth control' and 'the pill' were used synonymously and interchangeably in the debate. As Republicans spoke out against the contraceptive methods they associated with abortion - hormonal contraceptives and, less frequently, the IUD – the fervency of support for the pill and its derivatives (the implant, ring, patch, injection and hormonal IUD) increased.

Planned Parenthood and the mainstream women's health movement leapt to the defense of hormonal birth control, arguing that these methods are used not only for contraception but also to regulate periods, alleviate cramps and prevent acne. The drugs' benefits were talked up until they were claimed to be tantamount to cancer immunizations. The pill, in all its forms, was reiterated as a wonder drug and beyond criticism.

Bayer set about settling the 10,000 lawsuits of women who have taken Yaz and Yasmin and their families. The company is currently providing each woman who has suffered with injuries from blood clots and the families of those women that have died with hundreds of thousands of dollars in compensation. The first 500 cases addressed took a total of $110 million in payouts.

It wasn't just the older, the overweight or the understood 'at-risk' involved in these lawsuits, a large proportion were the young, fit and healthy women who had taken Yaz or Yasmin. These women had wanted clear skin or to lose a few pounds and, seeing as they were taking oral contraceptives anyway, thought these brands provided an amazing added bonus. One case described to me by a lawyer representing many of the plaintiffs involved a 20 year-old woman who had been training to be an Olympic skier when she started taking Yaz. She developed a blood clot that resulted in injuries that will prevent her from ever skiing again.

In the midst of the furor over the religious Right's anti-contraception agenda, US liberal pundit Rachel Maddow wrote an op-ed for *The Washington Post* in which she reported anxiously that Republican groups were marching with signs that read "The Pill Kills." Maddow was clearly unaware of the mounting lawsuits against Bayer.

Concerns over access had completely cancelled out issues of safety.

Of course, it is not solely the responsibility of the religious Right that there is so little interest in the women injured by these pills nor is this the product of the avid passion of the Left. There are clearly other equally oppressive forces at work unconnected to religion or conservativism, women's rights or liberalism. In the UK and Europe both conservative strains of religion and the pharmaceutical industry have a looser grip and yet the pill is raised just as high on a pedestal.

Should we consider that use of the pill for pregnancy

prevention, let alone acne or PMS, might still today, as women's health activist Barbara Seaman wrote in her radical women's health book *The Doctors' Case Against the Pill*, be "like tinkering with nuclear bombs to fight off the common cold"?

In 1969, when the book was published, the Congressional Nelson Pill Hearings saw women's health activists protest the lack of anecdotal evidence taken into account from the women who had actually used the pill and suffered as a result from the major depression, blood clots and many other illnesses it caused. Women's experiences were dismissed in favor of the scientific evidence provided by the male representatives of pharmaceutical companies and the proposals of those involved in programs for population control.

The FDA investigation into Yaz and Yasmin is a watershed moment in the history of the pill, and yet women do not know, were not told and or did not want to talk about it.

The popular, soft-feminism espousing website *Jezebel* was one the three media outlets that did discuss the investigation. The *Jezebel* writer reported the events under the headline: "New FDA Decisions Don't Mean Birth Control Is Killing You." The message was that open discussion of the risks should be suppressed, as it would cause a surge in unwanted pregnancies. The writer took the paternalistic tone of much contemporary feminist discussion of contraception in the US that treats women as though they were hysterics unable to handle the responsibility and complexity involved in truly informed consent. Truths and half-truths are manipulated to produce nothing less than propaganda for hormonal contraceptives. Any criticism is considered irresponsible, playing into the hands of those on the Right who want to see them banned. Yet neither side of the debate wants to talk honestly.

The pill is the sacred cow of the medical industry and protected defensively by those advocating for women. The pharmaceutical industry receives free advertising from those who claim to be working in women's best interests.

The FDA decision provided support for Bayer's choice to make settlements out of court. A lawyer privy to the confidential files of the Bayer Corporation admitted that just about anything would be done by the company's defense team to keep them from entering a trial and being forced to expose all records. Settlements kept Kessler's findings on the stealth marketing and the hidden research out of the spotlight.

Would we be foolish to assume the lies stopped with what we know, with just these brands of oral contraceptive or with this one pharmaceutical company?

Representatives from four women's health groups including Our Bodies Ourselves and the National Women's Health Network got together some months later to write a letter suggesting the question asked by the FDA of the advisory board was too vague to illicit a clear and certain response. The board members were asked to compare the risks of drospirenone-containing pills to the risks involved in pregnancy. The representatives argued it would be more logical to ask for a considered comparison of these drugs with other brands of oral contraceptives that are available to women. If that discussion were had, they stated, then drugs like Yaz and Yasmin would have surely been taken off the market. They are, after all, less safe than the many other pills that are equally effective at achieving their approved and paramount use of pregnancy prevention.

I believe it would be more appropriate to compare the risks of these drugs to non-hormonal methods of contraception.

In the few media reports it was argued that when compared to the risk of blood clot development associated with pregnancy, the risk produced by taking any oral contraceptive, including Yasmin or Yaz, is of little concern. This is misleading in that it suggests there are only two states in which young women can choose to live: on birth control pills or pregnant. Non-hormonal birth control methods hold no increased risk of blood clots and few side effects, if any. Some of these alternatives are equally effective in preventing pregnancy as oral contraceptives, and some even more so in practice. Such a comparison would obviously put the statistics on the risks in starker relief.

Although the women's health groups confronted the FDA, they chose to work with the pharmaceutical industry, rather than against its power.

The representatives told the FDA they believe "lives will be saved" if these brands are no longer on the market. They asked that the FDA "get back to the arc of history and progress that protects women while supporting their contraceptive needs," suggesting this decision was merely a blip on an otherwise uninterrupted curve of moral, uncorrupted action.

However, their flattery didn't get them far, as the FDA did not reconsider the conclusion. As the pills' effectiveness in pregnancy prevention was no more significant than any other oral contraceptive were they saying that other benefits seen as specific to these drugs - such as acne treatment, PMDD alleviation and prevention of bloating - were of such importance as to cancel out the high increase in risk of serious physical injury? Acne and bloating can be treated effectively without drugs. The diagnosis of PMDD is still controversial amongst those involved with the Diagnostic and Statistical Manual of Mental Disorders (DSM) and even then supposedly affects just eight percent of women.

Similarly the benefit gained from oral contraceptives in their prescription for potentially serious issues such as endometriosis and PCOS, which are suffered by around ten percent of women, are not specific to drugs containing drospirenone.

Why is it that we hear so little criticism of the pill coming from the side of the pro-choice, sex positive, feminist and liberal?

Dissenting voices that do suggest the pill may still hold health issues are systematically undermined as fear mongering or as sprung from a spurious anti-female agenda. Women's own experiences are ignored or derided as rare and tangential. The reasons for this are, I believe, ingrained in historical and social concepts of women and women's bodies. The narrowing of the narrative stems from how women see themselves and the ways in which they are willing to change themselves to please.

The support for women using hormonal contraceptives is built into the structure of our society. There are large-scale ideological, economical and social forces at work.

When I first began writing about my experience and investigating the pill's impact on women's health I regularly reiterated a disclaimer that I hoped would allow my voice to be heard above the din of denial. I am not a Catholic, I would say, I am not anti-contraception, pro-life or a frigid man-hater. I use condoms, spermicide and the fertility awareness method. I am a feminist.

In this culture it is not easy to find footing between the misogyny of the religious Right and the feminist agenda with its own brand of misogyny, but I believe it is a position worth fighting for. The silencing of honest discussion causes many women to suffer unnecessarily. It wasn't until I stopped taking the pill that I developed the needed energy, motivation and clarity of thought to express why I had to stop and to question why it had taken me so long to make that decision.

Section One: In The Habit

"The issue was whether any woman would take a pill every day to prevent the chance she might get pregnant. They believed no one's going to do that, not when they're not even sick, and they're not even sick!" - James Balog, Merck Pharmaceuticals (*The Doctor's Case Against The Pill*, Barbara Seaman)

"I'd been on the pill for ten years, having originally been prescribed it for my teenage acne, then I carried on taking it for extra double strength contraception. Then, when I was twenty-six, I suddenly decided I'd had enough and stopped taking it. I felt like a cloud had been lifted, as if before I had been living in black and white and now I was living in full color. I know this sounds mad, but it felt like I was just more alive. I also had these feelings of being more womanly, more attractive and more sexual and sexually powerful. People commented that I had blossomed. I felt more confident, my creativity overflowed in my work as a textile designer. I'd been awakened creatively. The emotional changes I felt when I came off the pill were huge, I would go so far as to say life changing. That is how I would describe the experience of coming off the pill - an awakening" - Laura

Who am I when I'm not on the pill?

I took the pill even when it wasn't for the purpose of preventing pregnancy. Throughout my teens, which I spent at an all-girls grammar school, I wasn't having sex. When I eventually did have sex the pill was my back-up method and used with condoms. Taking the pill each morning was an unthinking habit that began when my mother took me to the family doctor, having decided it was the right time to start. I had two older sisters; both on the pill, and my mother had the ingrained fear of unwanted pregnancy plus the sensibility of someone who came of age as the pill arrived.

I would not say I chose to take the pill but I can not say I protested or that I would have not made the decision independently. It felt like a right of passage, a kind of gateway to adulthood. If you were not having sex, taking the pill was the next best thing. I had not particularly minded the heavy, painful periods I had endured for the previous three years. They got me out of the gym classes I hated and allowed me to lie down in the school's quiet, dark sick room instead of taking a math test.

I accepted taking the pill in the same way that I accepted that I would go to school each day or take my exams or apply for college. No other options were discussed so taking the pill became something I just had to do, something every woman eventually did. I had no clue how the pill worked and I had no clue how my body worked. My science classes covered the minimum details of the menstrual cycle but I didn't ask for the connection between that and the pink packets of tablets I kept in my make up bag and that information was not offered.

Studies show that young women are less likely to get pregnant using a combination of condoms and spermicide than the pill because they will use them with more regularity. This is partly because condoms have a clear connection to their purpose. We know how they prevent pregnancy and so when taught to use both properly the effectiveness rate is high. The pill is prescribed carelessly and taken thoughtlessly. It is prescribed to teens who do not have a real understanding of its actions.

Women are not trusted by their doctors with more information than is viewed as strictly necessary. This tablet will "regulate" your periods, is often the first description of the pill's impact we hear and it is the first half-truth told to women about how the pill works.

I used condoms when I was supposed to, but when I was

supposed to forgo them I didn't. I didn't trust the pill to do what it was made to do. I felt it was essential to take the pill regardless of my decision to continue conscientiously using condoms in my first committed relationship.

I knew that my reliance on this drug extended beyond contraception. I understood that taking the pill was what I had to do as a woman, like shaving my legs or wearing make-up.

Even when I began to suspect the pill was making me ill, I still found it immensely difficult to stop performing the ritual. Making the connection between my physical and emotional health issues and the pill was not simple or easy. I blamed everything but the pill for a long time.

My struggle with stopping made me think that I had a psychological, if not a physical, dependency on this drug. I had developed a reliance on what the pill was doing for me. In order to stop I had to unravel this complex relationship with a medication that had been at my side for over a decade. The pill had been assimilated into my sense of self; it had become a part of my life and of me. It was an adaptation that had seen me through my transition from girl to woman.

I was, I felt, addicted to the pill.

The crux was that I knew who I was on the pill and I didn't know whom I'd be if I came off. At that time, I hoped that I would be happier, relaxed, and healthier, but my pre-pill years were a long time ago. I had started on it before I even had an idea of who I might be; back when I was still physically and mentally coming into form as a young woman.

Yasmin ruined me, and retrospectively I could see how all of the brands of pill I had taken had had an insidious effect on my body that wore me down and eroded my emotional and physical strength. I could also see how certain brands might have caused me to react in ways similar to Yasmin. The realizations came slowly.

It wasn't until some two years off the pill I recalled that my inability to sit in the exam hall at school without a panic attack had come about in the first year of the pill. From that point on, through college, I requested to be sat at a desk in the back corner of the room so I would not feel trapped. I had gone away to college and, depressed and anxious, asked to transfer to my hometown university within a month. It was an experience that seemed so out-of-character to friends, family and myself. To think about how a drug may have impacted on my experience of events big and small makes me angry.

I wonder – what would I have done if I'd not been on the pill?

Many of the women who went through what I did on Yasmin or Yaz found it ended their relationship. When I explained my Yasmin-stoked behavior to my boyfriend, he related the realizations I was having to his struggle to stop smoking cigarettes. It was an analogy that resonated with me as I'd seen how stopping and restarting cigarettes changed his personality. I got that the easily irritated, emotionally-wrought, foggy-headed, out-of-it feelings that taking the pill gave me were similar to the way he said he felt in a state of consistent nicotine withdrawal.

After reading my blog a friend wrote to me and expanded on this thought. When a person smokes for long enough, he speculated, they become "a smoker" and as such "a biological extension of a medicinal parasite." Smoking, he argued, hijacks your personality and your sense of self. The smoking becomes a routine you have to stick to and as you go about that routine the chemicals meddle with your emotions.

When a woman takes the pill for however many months, years or decades she is unlikely to see herself as 'a pill-taker.' She is unlikely to consider taking the pill in the same way she might think about taking another drug, like painkillers, every day.

There are few drugs, although the list is ever expanding, that people who are not sick take every day for large portions of their lifetimes.

The marketing technique Bayer adopted is known as the

"Virginia Slims model" of advertising. The cigarette brand's commercials co-opted the language of the women's liberation movement to appeal directly to young women. This focus gained them a significant increase in profits. Smoking these cigarettes was linked to ideas of glamour, modernity, independence and attractiveness. The adverts went so far as to suggest it was a woman's duty to honor her hard-won independence by smoking Virginia Slims.

Every time I had a health issue caused by the pill my doctor would suggest I just try another brand. The complaints I took to my doctor prior to Yasmin ranged from migraines to constant bleeding to nausea.

Like many young women, I was petrified of pregnancy. I believe the intensity of this anxiety had much to do with the length of time I took the pill. Through a decade of pill taking I was completely cut off from any sense of my body's true physicality. In fact, I had come to fear the potential of my body. My fertility was something I felt needed to be fought constantly. I was suspicious of my body's capabilities and felt they needed to be restrained at any cost. I had no idea how my body would feel if I were pregnant, or how it would feel if I were not. I only knew of one state, that produced by the pill. If I used condoms I could see that they had worked, but the pill left me constantly wondering if the day I forgot to take the tablet until the evening would be my undoing.

When I came off the pill for a couple of months after using Yasmin and switching to Femodette I was saying to myself that being on the pill was making me very sick, but that I still felt that getting pregnant would be worse. I assumed that my only sensible contraceptive choice was the pill. It was the pill or nothing. I had received this message loud and clear from all the parties invested in preventing me from getting pregnant – my parents, my doctor, and my friends. If the condom broke, I took the morning-after pill too, something I did twice during my decade on the pill.

Over the years I felt no connection between my self and my body, between my self and the world around me, between my femaleness and myself. I was blocked somehow, cut-off and isolated. My instincts, both physically manifested and emotional, were non-existent.

When I came off the pill it was like the lights got switched back on for me. I soon had the capacity to feel deeply and fully in a way I had not felt for many years and with that I had the capacity to truly connect.

When I started taking the pill again it was because my life had started to change very quickly. When my routine was threatened, the pill ritual seemed like a reassurance and a comfort. I was all too ready to hear that I ought to stay on the pill. Going back on the pill felt like taking control at a time when I felt things were spinning out of control in the rest of my life. I didn't believe in my ability to cope with the necessary upheaval I was facing. The feeling was similar to how I felt the need to police my eating habits during times of high stress in order to experience a sense of order in my life. I felt uncertain about the depth and complexity of my newly awakened emotions and thoughts. My own experience, my own desires were not stronger than the pressure I felt internally and externally to continue with my pill taking.

When I finally came off the pill for good, I had months of intense withdrawal. It was a state similar to my worst times on Yasmin. A friend who came off the pill a year prior described her experience to me when I was in the midst of this experience and was unbelieving that this could be down to oral contraceptives. She said she had experienced a strongly a feeling of "intuition gone wrong" during her withdrawal, a creeping paranoia that built into dread. I felt at that time, as she had been through, that I should be wary and suspicious of all that had before brought comfort and happiness, especially people close to me. My body was flooded with chemical messages of danger telling me to hide or run as my endocrine system rebooted.

I kept one packet of Femodette pills on hand just incase I changed my mind, but the more I read and wrote about the pill the clearer it became that I could never take it again.

When a woman takes the pill for over a decade events will occur to make her rightfully sad and angry. I have frequently been told I shouldn't blame any changes to my physical or mental health on the pill just because I happened to be taking it when they came about.

During that time of withdrawal, when I was thinking about the difference between my mood changes on the pill and my mood changes off the pill I would visualize myself as a boat tied to a dock. On and off the pill the sea can get rough and choppy, but when I was on the pill that anchor was no longer there and the boat would be pummeled and pushed out to sea. Now I am off the pill however rough the sea gets there is still that anchor, the mooring to that solid land that is tangible.

I was sick, and then, I was well. That this is not enough evidence of the pill's impact reveals so much about why women are encouraged to take this drug in the first place.

In writing about my experience I came to understand that taking the pill was bound up with how I felt about myself and about being a woman. I was a "pill-taker" for a decade and when I came off it was life changing.

The pill-takers

The pill's rise in popularity was rapid. Between 1962 and 1969, the number of women taking the pill rose from 50,000 to one million. In the US, 1.2 million women used the pill within two years of its launch.

Today eighty percent of women will take the birth control pill at some point during their lifetimes. Three hundred million women have used the pill across the globe; one hundred million are currently taking the tablets each day. Three and a half million women in the UK and fourteen million women in the US are on the pill. Twenty-eight percent of all of the women that are using birth control in the US take the pill, which makes it the most popular non-permanent form of contraception.

Sixty-four percent of women between twenty and twenty-four in the UK use the pill. Fifty percent of women under age twenty-five use the pill in the US – fifty-three percent of those are aged fifteen to nineteen and forty seven percent of those are aged twenty to twenty-four.

Tens of millions more use the derivatives of the pill, known as LARCs or long-acting reversible contraceptives (such as the injection Depo Provera, the implant NexPlanon, the vaginal ring Nuvaring and the hormonal IUD Mirena). A US federal study from the National Center for Health Statistics found that the use of long-acting hormonal methods has increased by seventy-five percent since 1995, and IUD use (the study did not differentiate between the hormonal Mirena or the non-hormonal copper IUD ParaGard) had increased six hundred percent since 2006. However, oral contraceptives still dominate as these methods only retain a relatively small percentage of birth control use – seven percent of women overall use the patch or ring and only five percent use the IUD.

Taking hormonal contraceptives is an experience shared by the majority of women.

Only forty-two percent of American women on the pill admit to using it solely for contraceptive purposes. Fifty percent say they want to regulate their periods and are prescribed the pill for this reason first.

More and more of these women will take the pill continuously from mid-teens to menopause with breaks for children.

Studies suggest that half of women on the pill are aware of suffering from depression and anxiety. A 1998 study from the

University of North Carolina, a 2001 Kinsey Institute study, a 2005 Monash University study, and 2008 Lakehead University research all show dissatisfaction with the pill is widespread as a result specifically of its negative impact on emotional well-being.

The survival factor or drop-out rate in studies suggest that there are a large number of women who stop taking the pill after a few months due to intolerable side effects. There are not many published research studies into the emotional impact of hormonal contraceptives considering the number of years the drug has been in existence, and even fewer that are released and published in the mainstream media.

In contrast, the World Health Organization held a six-country study into the potential impact of a male hormonal contraceptive on men's well-being and sexuality and the possibility of such a drug's acceptance and success. A drug that prevents a man from producing sperm is seen as more radical than a drug that prevents women from releasing eggs. The WHO study suggested there is concern over how a male hormonal contraceptive would impact attributes of masculinity.

It is often hard to discern the onset of insidious depression and anxiety. As they develop, they become part of life and a person gets used to living with feelings that seem to have always been there. If a woman takes the pill for years she may not be consciously aware of its impact on her mental health. She may think she feels a certain way "naturally," that it is just in her character to be nervous or to cry at the slightest thing. She may assume her problems are due to her circumstances. If a woman has taken the pill since her teens it is even harder for her to know if her emotional outlook has changed.

Health problems caused by hormonal contraceptives can appear a few months, a few years or longer into use as each woman processes the synthetic chemicals differently.

Yet all women will be changed by these drugs.

As a woman's body changes so does her reaction to the pill.

The pill's repression of vital bodily functions that leads to ill health can build in such a way that years later a woman becomes very sick but can not make the connection.

Of course, all drugs that we take have side effects but few are taken every day, for years, by healthy people.

At the time of the pill's release, there was an expectation that it would be taken for no more than a few years. Women got married and started families earlier and they only took it when in a relationship. The pill was a form of contraception first and foremost although it was prescribed for what were called "menstrual disorders" at the time. Although mainly prescribed to married women, the pill was advertised as an accessory for the young, sexy, and modern woman. It was not, however, seen as the cure-all it is today.

The impact of the pill on women's health has never been studied over a length of time that is equal to the number of years that many women take the drug. Nor has there been research into the impact on children born to women using hormonal birth control.

The diaphragm was at the time of the pill's release a popular contraceptive method for the independent and single woman, but by 1965 the pill was the most popular form of birth control in the US.

The pill wipes out all the ups and downs, Gray areas and subtleties that the female body's hormone cycle produces monthly. Emotional experience is flattened and there are studies that reflect this, albeit in a positive light. The studies read an absence of emotional reaction to exterior forces as a desirable and positive affect. The researchers work from the standpoint that women do not enjoy their monthly ups and downs. When the pill stops the downs, it also stops the ups – it does not differentiate. Women are told that the pill causes their body to mimic pregnancy when in fact the opposite is true, it causes the body to maintain very low levels of hormones.

The pill is as intrinsic to Western patriarchal capitalist culture as it is to the lives of millions of women. What would our society be without the pill?

Despite the pill being a part of a vast number of women's lives and taking the pill a collectively shared experience of so many writings on female sexuality, both female body politics and female psychology fail to draw this experience into the discussion. In feminist theory the pill is either considered an inarguable, intrinsic good or it is a non-issue.

We can read about how the release of the pill changed the fight for women's liberation or changed women's position in society, but not how it changed women.

Old myths as new fictions

In the 1800s doctors would advise that women who were difficult, argumentative or too overtly sexual should be given an ovariectomy. The removal of the ovaries was believed to cure women of these problems. They became, as Barbara Ehrenreich and Deirdre English describes in *For Her Own Good*, "orderly, industrious and cleanly." An ovariectomy was referred to then as female castration.

The pill is essentially a modern version of this procedure; its aim is to "shut down" the ovaries. The aim of preventing pregnancy is brought about through crude and aggressive means. The ovaries are shut down long-term even though women are fertile for just a few days of each month. The highest level of synthetic hormones necessary to shut down the ovulatory process in all women is used. It is a one-size-fits-all method of treatment, just as an ovariectomy was considered a cure-all because it combated a whole variety of singularly female ailments.

The 'rest cure' was also often prescribed for women perceived as difficult during this same era. In the Victorian-era there was an epidemic of "sickness" in women. Middle class women were prevented from working, reading or learning. All attention was placed on their bodies. The fainting, weak and child-like woman was held up as the standard of attractiveness: imagine it to be the 'heroin chic' of the 1990s. Women would actually drink vinegar and arsenic in order to make themselves sick and achieve this level of beauty.

Ehrenreich and English speculate that women were aware that they could avoid being forced to bear more children if they took to their beds with sicknesses for long lengths of time. Being sick could be manipulated to be a woman's source of power and control over her situation.

The uterus was understood to be the central controlling organ for the rest of a woman's body. Medical practitioners believed that the uterus worked in competition with the brain. These two organs could not function harmoniously. The uterus prevented rational and logical thought and caused mental and intellectual weakness. This fundamental problem within their bodies caused women to become sick.

Therefore all women were inescapably, inherently ill as a result of their own biology. Femaleness was a mental illness that required constant management.

However, the medical industry was faced with a dilemma of their own making by this diagnosis. Women were required to be pregnant, but could not if they were deemed sick. The concept of hysteria became the answer to this quandary. If a woman could be proven hysterical rather than truly sick she could continue to have children. At that time children were the main focus of the medical field and the act of raising a child was elevated to the highest level of social importance.

Child rearing became so important in fact that it needed to be taken out of the hands of women. A pregnant woman, it was believed, was under the influence of the "horror of being female," a psychosis that made her untrustworthy and dangerous. With this reasoning, doctors could justify intervention in the child rearing process although it had previously mainly been the domain of midwives and female relations.

Later in the 1950s, as Enrenreich and English describe, when the consumer economy took hold, women had a certain power as the most influential consumers. The economy is driven best by the manifestation of traits of selfishness, ruthlessness and individualism. Yet women were relegated to home life where they took care of their children and undertook their wifely duties with an apparent selfless sense of purpose. These women did not fit into the boundaries of the capitalist-inspired view of human nature. To explain the conflict, medical authorities branded women masochists. It was masochism that drove them to sacrifice their independence to their family. Self-denial in an economy thriving on instant-gratification and consumption was a disease.

Sex hormones were discovered in the 1920s but synthetic hormones were developed in Nazi Germany, as Barbara Seaman first highlighted. Bayer Schering Corp – now Bayer – developed synthetic estrogen and experimented on Jewish prisoners in the hope of sterilizing them. They found that although women stopped menstruating they were not made permanently infertile. This became an important part of the process of developing the pill.

The medical industry in the 1950s blamed menstrual problems and infertility on "incomplete feminization." If women were unhappy in their prescribed role they were "rejecting their femininity." Menstrual cycle and fertility issues were therefore purely psychosomatic. Women were told that if only they embraced the femaleness of their biology they would not experience problems.

Misogynistic medical understanding of female biology was used as justification for women's oppression. Embracing this view of female biology required embracing and accepting the oppression. Women were likely to do anything to avoid being confronted by their own femaleness when it was defined in such limited and negative terms.

It could be said that women were rejecting the concept of femininity presented to them by society, a concept they had no part in creating. Their unhappiness with their standing in society was protest and not pathology. Menstrual health issues and infertility were not self-inflicted and psychosomatic, although such issues may have been worsened by chronic stress. By blaming women the medical establishment was divorcing women from their own bodies and making the female body an object of and a source for fear and oppression. If they had physical health issues women were told to blame themselves and their faulty, weak bodies.

The "psychology" of the ovary and uterus was a rationalization for the social inferiority of women to men. These ideas were still very much alive in medical journals and doctor's practices when the pill was created and are still in circulation today.

When the pill was released it provided the opportunity to silence these rationalizations that had plagued women for so long. The pill shut down the troublesome organs. Without these organs weakening their bodies and minds the argument for keeping them out of the workplace and the realm of men had shaky foundation. It became a necessary part of the progress of women's liberation that women deny female biology. Women were needed to work for the economy by this time and instead of overthrowing the misogynistic medical understanding of women's bodies, women took the pill that provided an easy answer to the conflict.

Without their ovaries intervening women could be viewed as "industrious." They could be seen as more like men. The pill helped women fit into the male-dominated social structure and economy.

Far from being a revolutionary moment in history, the invention and prescription of the pill fit very neatly into the developing consumer-based capitalist economy. To sustain consumption women also needed to work and make money. The medical establishment had proclaimed women incapable of working alongside men, but the pill gave them an escape route.

In 1969 feminist writer Clare Boothe Luce said, "Modern woman is at last free, as a man is free, to dispose of her own body, to earn a living…to try a successful career."

"Dispose" is a critical choice of word. By one definition it is saying women could arrange their bodies in an orderly fashion; by another it is saying women could transfer control of their bodies to others, and by a third definition it is saying women could "deal" with their bodies conclusively. All three actions are achieved by taking the pill.

Women were, of course, working already and effectively using condoms or the diaphragm to prevent pregnancy, but the pill gave that needed push towards social acceptance of this new course of life for them. The medical industry still believed that female biology incapacitated women both physically and mentally. The invention of the pill was not a sign of the medical industry working in the best interests of women; it was a demonstration of the misogyny at the foundation of their practices.

Equally, women's acceptance of the pill was not a sign of their liberation but an illustration of the internalization of this misogyny. Women were happy to medicate themselves, because they had been told for so long that they were sick. If that sickness was their responsibility then it was their responsibility to cure it, by taking the pill.

Women would still bleed during their week off of the pill every month. The medical cycle was planned out as a marketing tool. It was also necessary for men and society at large to accept women taking the pill and a fake period made the pill appear more natural. Women could be equal in society, but not too equal. The fake 'period' would not be incapacitating but it was a reminder of women's inherent weakness. In the present day, we have no need for such a marketing tool.

In this way, the pill is a rejection of femaleness. In swallowing the tablets women are swallowing the negative connotations that are attached to female biology.

The pill allowed for doctors to extend their intervention from child rearing to fertility, and medicate women from their teenage years to menopause.

Feminism has established itself as a reaction to the assertion that biology is destiny. This reaction is founded on the acceptance and internalization of the misogynistic medical ideology.

In 1953 Dr Katherina Dalton identified and coined the term premenstrual syndrome or PMS as a hormone-related phase of health issues experienced during the fourteen days before menstruation. Published in 1978, her bestselling book *Once a Month: The Premenstrual Syndrome Handbook* claims that PMS "threatens the very foundations of society." Decades later Karen Houppert, author of *The Curse: Confronting the Last Unmentionable Taboo: Menstruation*, suggested that during World War Two the inherent weakness of women was played down purposefully. Women were required to take over traditionally male jobs when men were drafted to fight. Yet when the men returned, women needed to be hustled back into the kitchen quickly and quietly. The fact that women had proven themselves to be equally capable was suppressed. She suggests the debate about the negative impact of PMS or 'unpredictable' hormones on women has resurfaced since then at the most opportune times.

The existence of PMDD has never been proven scientifically, although it is registered as a mental illness with a potential 200 broad symptoms ranging from nervousness to anger to stress.

In comparison, in contemporary society PMS is blamed for all manner of female-defined emotions. Recent research argues that women could experience PMS symptoms at any time during the month, not just before menstruation. A woman is said to be PMS-ing if she is disagreeable in any way.

Dr Dalton argued in her book that although PMS caused problems for women it also cost American society eight percent of the total wage bill. When experiencing PMS women could not be trusted with the simplest tasks, not even taking care of their children. A woman's menstrual cycle was everyone's business. Women's emotions were seen as a threat to society. Just as hysteria was a threat to the continuation of society in preventing women from having children, PMS might cause women to harm children.

Even if women were rightfully angry to be relegated once again to the sphere of female work, their anger was quickly reduced to a symptom of this syndrome. Psychologist Paula Caplan remarks that this diagnosis amounted to the medical authorities saying to women – "We'll believe what you women tell us about how you're feeling but you've got to let us call you mentally ill."

Within this narrative the pill could be understood as freeing women from the tyranny of their troubled emotional states and allowing them to become more consistent and stable. Yasmin and Yaz were promoted as cures for anxiety, moodiness and PMDD. Stabilizing moods is even more prevalent in the pill promotion today than when it was first released. Biological, physical and mental consistency and stability were considered important requirements for entry into the working world with its repetitious, rigid schedule and myriad unrewarding roles.

There are parallels and intersections between the development of the feminine hygiene industry and the progression of the pill. The tampon hides the period, but the pill gets rid of the period altogether.

Our relationship to the pill is inseparable from our relationship to menstruation. Brands of the pill such as Seasonique and Lybrel are promoted on the basis of letting women have just four fake periods a year. They are first and foremost menstrual suppressants with the added benefit of pregnancy prevention. These brands were advertised heavily on US television channels like *Spiked* that are directed towards men.

Women are asked by their doctor how many times a year they want to have their period and many respond that they never want to have another period, without knowing what they are throwing away. Menstruation and ovulation are not connected in this dialogue. Menstruation is subsumed by the fake period, which can be easily disregarded as purely an old-fashioned marketing invention. Ovulation is presumed unnecessary unless a woman wants to get pregnant.

For the pill to gain more of the women's health market negative views on menstruation had to be perpetuated and elaborated. The feminine hygiene and the pharmaceutical industry did not have to create this issue, only draw on ideas already present in the ideology and repackage them for new generations. As the popularity of the pill increased, and therefore more women had shorter and lighter fake periods or no fake period at all, the feminine hygiene industry developed new problems that could be solved by their products. Women should not sweat, urinate, blow their noses or emit any bodily secretions, but especially menstrual blood. The development of sanitary pads for daily use and not just during menstruation is one illustration of the strategy. The cervical mucus produced during the cycle that can be used as a clear sign of the window of fertility, or be a marker of infection, is drawn into a bleached pad and treated as a dirty secretion.

As Houppert reports a sign on the wall of the foyer of the Tambrands factory reads, "If it ain't broke, fix it anyway."

There is much great writing available on society's menstrual taboo and not enough space to cover this at length here except to say that our cultural view of menstruation has acted as a catalyst for our eager uptake of hormonal contraceptives. We have been told for decades that periods are unfeminine, unattractive and gross and that having a period is shameful and unbearable. Chris Bobel has explored this topic in her excellent book, *New Blood: Third Wave Feminism and the Politics of Menstruation*.

The Nelson Pill Hearings made women implicit in their medicalization. Women demanded that the pill be improved and they demanded that information be provided in inserts. The pharmaceutical companies had to approve the improvements if they were to keep selling the pill. Just as women had supported the development of drugs to ease pain during birth, they supported the development of the pill. After this, women's support of hormonal contraceptives only increased. A relatively brief period of suspicion gave way to women taking the pill in higher numbers than ever before.

Do we feel the same way now about hormonal contraceptives as we did then?

If we can accept that the release of the pill was a necessary social event, we can consider that it has now outlived that necessity. We could agree that the pill has no place in modern medicine.

It is as we are changing from a child to an adult that women are prescribed the pill. Teenage girls' reproductive systems are shut down before they are fully developed. Their endocrine system is manipulated as they go through volatile puberty. Hormonal contraceptives are prescribed to teenagers as a treatment for normal short-term symptoms of bodily transition – the heavy periods, cramps and acne. When you take hormonal contraceptives as a teen it impacts on your developing libido and displaces your sexuality. The heavy periods stop, skin becomes clearer, hair less greasy and the transition to adulthood is sped along, missing out some vital steps along the way. In the US teen girls are given Accutane for acne and, because the effects of the drug on a developing embryo are unknown, the birth control pill at the same time. It is medically understood that teen girls go through a time during which their bodies grow accustomed to the menstrual cycle and this maturation and adjustment is what causes heavy bleeding and cramps.

The pill and its derivatives has become a short cut to the concept of womanhood.

Do you want to take the pill?

The discussion of the pill in mainstream media is bogged in the traditional misogyny found in the history of the medical industry. In today's publications we read that depression when on the pill is the result of a woman mourning her inability to get pregnant, we see menstruation classed as dangerous and hear a call for the uterus and ovaries to be kept quiet.

Doctors defend their choice to not inform women of side effects with the claim that they want to avoid putting ideas into the heads of those prone to irrational thoughts. Women are told that they must protect their fertility and that unchecked menstruation is disabling. Tabloid stories about women who choose to pursue a career by becoming infertile or women thwarted by their biological clock are steeped in Victorian-era based beliefs about women's capacity for work.

Emily Martin, in *The Woman in the Body*, compares the language used to describe the male reproductive system with that used to describe menstruation and ovulation. She argues that negative phrasing is utilized for female biology – words such as "ceasing," "dying" and "losing." Whereas the development of sperm production is described as an amazing feat of nature.

Martin views the negative associations of female reproduction through the ideology of capitalism. Capitalism demands productivity in its workers. Women's bodies are not productive when they're not pregnant; in fact their functions are based in waste, waste of the egg and waste of the uterine lining.

Martin asks, "How do women respond to scientific metaphors

about their bodies? Do they accept them as natural and as women's rightful due or resign themselves to tolerating them? Or do they fight them as deep and sinister threats to their existence?"

Women often discuss menstruation and birth as happening to them, rather than as part of them and their experience. Martin remarks that women often see their self as separate to their body. Women's central image is that "your body is something your self has to adjust to or cope with" and therefore, Martin concludes, "your body needs to be controlled by your self."

Martin explores the idea that women did not fit into the structure of the jobs that were open to them in industrialized society. These jobs most often required monotony, routine and repetition. Although in reality no more suited to men than they were women, it was women that were judged as innately unable to succeed in such positions due on the constantly changing and supposedly unpredictable nature of their physical state.

As Martin states, "Women were perceived as malfunctioning and their hormones out of balance," especially when experiencing PMS and menstruation, "rather than the organization of society and work perceived as in need of transformation to demand less constant discipline and productivity."

The rigidity of society was forcefully imposed on women as it was on men. For all, both men and women, it is inhumane but it was women that were required to adapt in a more dramatic and overt way. Men are viewed as naturally given to the industrious and disciplined way of life demanded of them and the structure of society is built on these assumed capabilities.

If we admit that women do change through the month, that we do menstruate, experience PMS, have differing moods week to week, we fear that this admission will be used as justification for negative judgment.

Martin counters the feminist refrain of "biology is not destiny"; "I think the way out of this bind is to focus on women's experiential statements – that they function differently during certain days. We could then perhaps hear these statements not as warnings of the flaws inside women that need to be fixed, but as insights into flaws in society that need to be addressed."

The idea that men are otherwise unchanging is falsified. Men also experience hormonal changes with studies suggesting they experience a cycle daily that is equivalent to the monthly cycle of women as well as changes in hormone levels across their lifetimes.

Women's "experiential statements" as Martin describes them are often silenced in the discourse surrounding hormonal contraceptives. It is a betrayal of the feminist cause to speak out with openness about the side effects of the pill.

When Yaz and Yasmin were released the marketing strategy co-opted the idea of word of mouth. In a commercial women were seen passing along the "secret" of these new drugs with their host of beneficial yet superficial side effects. Receiving messages of increased physical attractiveness as the result of a drug that many women were using anyway, only a different brand, increased the transference of this experience from one woman to the next.

In the face of such powerful manipulation, what place does a skillfully worded informational insert have in women's decision-making process? The time of the Nelson Pill Hearings was a very different to today.

Naomi Wolf mentions the pill briefly in *The Beauty Myth*. She remarks that it was originally marketed as a drug to keep women "young, beautiful and sexy," concepts parallel to those promoted by Bayer through its contemporary advertising. Wolf quotes, in the context of the beauty industry, John Galbraith, "Behavior that is essential for economic reasons is transformed into social virtue."

Women who do not want to take the pill are treated as difficult and irresponsible. If they do not accept the pill they are ungrateful of the work of women in history and of the privilege afforded them.

Today the initial decision to take the pill is often made for teenage girls. Many of them do not reassess the decision independently until they are well into their twenties by which time their relationship to the drug and to their bodies is so complex as to potentially prevent them successfully coming off the pill. The choice to take the pill is fiercely protected and yet that choice is rarely autonomous and informed.

It is not active choice making, but passive acceptance.

Section Two: The Drug

"Never in history have so many individuals taken such potent drugs with so little information as to the actual and potential hazards. We are embarking on a massive endocrinologic experiment on millions of health women." Senator Gaylord Nelson, 1970 during the Nelson Pill Hearings (*The Doctor's Case Against the Pill*, Barbara Seaman)

"I stopped taking the pill because I was single and simply didn't feel like renewing my prescription. Within that same month or two I started feeling really positive, awake, and alive. It was so dramatic that people around me noticed the change. I eventually realized that this burst of joy, which has not subsided in the three years I have been off the pill, synced up with when I quit the pill. I had been depressed for so long that I did not even know I was depressed. I thought that I was just an unhappy person." - Kat

What you don't know...

When I asked Dr Peter Bowen-Simpkins, a gynecologist and spokesperson for the organization Wellbeing for Women, why GPs do not fully explain the pill's actions to their patients he replied, 'Why wouldn't you be satisfied with just knowing it stops you producing eggs so you don't get pregnant?'

The pill is often described as "regulating" periods. This piece of information, without context, is not just useless, but misleading. The pill does not regulate women's periods. That would mean that women on the pill continued to have periods, only more regularly spaced. The bleeding, or fake period, experienced when on the pill is a withdrawal bleed and not like menstruation in anything other than the appearance of blood.

The pill is designed to disrupt the endocrine system, which

regulates all hormonal systems in the body, including the sex hormones.

This means the pill exerts changes on every bodily system.

In a woman's reproductive hormone cycle huge hormonal fluctuations occur that have an impact on the whole body, right down to her sense of taste and smell. The pill causes hormone levels to mimic that of a menopausal woman and so a pill-taker has a similar set of potential health issues to a woman going through that stage in her life.

The sex hormone cycle regulates 150 bodily systems all of which are suppressed by hormonal contraceptives and all of which are interrelated to all other body systems (including the endocrine, neurologic and immunologic systems). Therefore hormonal contraceptives impact:

Energy levels
Memory and concentration
Motor coordination
Adrenalin levels
Pain threshold
Vitamin retention
Blood glucose levels
Thyroid and adrenal function
Sleep patterns
Body temperature
Skin color and texture
Brain wave patterns
Metabolism rate
Visual, auditory and olfactory acuity
Concentrations of vitamins
Immune system

Ovulation is triggered by fluctuations in sex hormones, but so are many other systems within the body. The pill interferes with the functioning of the monthly cycle of sex hormones in order to prevent ovulation and replaces it with a continuous flattened flow of synthetic estrogen and progesterone.

The stream of synthetic hormones does not function or fluctuate as the natural hormone cycle would and this change in function and levels of normal hormones through the month affects every system dependent on those natural hormones.

The ovaries are inextricably linked with the entire endocrine system. The hypothalamus, the pituitary gland, parathyroid, thyroid, adrenal gland and pancreas are all connected to the hormone-releasing ovaries and the rest of the body. The endocrine system is also inextricably linked to neurological and immunological functions.

The pill does not mimic a woman's natural cycle as we are often told – if it did then it would not prevent ovulation. During the natural cycle of hormones the level of estrogen will rise after menstruation until peaking just before ovulation. After ovulation the effect of estrogen is modified by levels of progesterone that are about ten times higher and remain so for approximately two weeks.

We hear much about "endocrine disrupters" today. Often they are discussed as found in plastics, pesticides, cleaning products, furniture and personal hygiene products and this knowledge has pushed people towards choosing chemical-free over chemical-saturated products.

Birth control pills are, by their very design, endocrine disruptors, but they are not mentioned alongside the shampoos and kitchen cleaners in this conversation.

People now make an effort to avoid potential endocrine disruptors, but they do not question taking the pill. Decreased or lost fertility is one of the impacts of endocrine disrupters that are talked about in the media and obviously this is a desired impact of the pill, but there is a range of other effects on the body not linked back to hormonal contraceptives. Often at the center of the voiced concern is the impact of endocrine disruptors on male fertility, although women take endocrine disruptors for this purpose.

The pill inhabits a blind spot when in comes to women's health.

Founder of Justisse and Director of Justisse Health Works For Women Geraldine Matus highlights, "I believe one of the easiest ways for the pharmaceutical companies to dupe women into thinking contraceptive endocrine disruptors are okay to use is by calling synthetic estrogens like estradiol by the name of estrogen. We need to call a spade a spade to begin to break the spell we are under with respect to the pill and her relatives."

Matus has worked has worked as a fertility awareness and birth control educator and holistic reproductive health practitioner for over thirty years. On our use of the term "the pill" to encompass all oral contraceptives, she says, "We euphemistically call this drug, an endocrine disrupter, "the pill" as if it were a pet or something innocuous. Using euphemistic terms for hormonal contraceptives creates a cognitive disconnect from the hard reality of us taking a drug that affects every system of our body."

Laura Eldridge writes in *In Our Control* about how the discussion of the impact of synthetic hormones from pharmaceuticals has been hijacked by the religious Right. They have made it into a stick to beat women who use hormonal contraceptives. She asks that we consider what impact pharmaceutical pollution as a whole has on the environment from all of the top selling; most used drugs that go through us and into our waters. Eldridge's mentor Barbara Seaman worked to raise awareness of impact of the pill as an endocrine disrupter in women's bodies, what she called "the elephant in the room."

When we discuss the endocrine disrupting chemicals in plastics or the meat we eat, the synthetic hormones we take over years en masse do not factor.

The most commonly prescribed pills are called combined, as

they contain both a synthetic estrogen and progesterone. The level of ethinyl estradiol (one of the synthetic estrogens) can range from 20mcg to 35mcg. A number of different types of progestin (the synthetic progesterone) are used across the brands. Doctors almost always recommend pills that are monophasic. Also available are synthetic progesterone-only pills, which have no synthetic estrogen content.

There are two groups of progestins – the first contains levonorgestrel and norethisterone. The pills with these elements are progesterone-dominant. The second group includes desogestrel, gestodene, norgestimate and drospirenone, progestins, which are used in estrogen-dominant pills, so-called because the ethinylestradiol is not acted on by the progestin. These are usually prescribed as the second choice if a woman complains of side effects from a pill containing one of the progestins that is in the first group. The progestin element of the brand Dianette, for example, is an anti-androgen (testosterone is an androgen) called cyproterone acetate and this is specifically prescribed for its suppression of testosterone. Testosterone levels play a part in acne production.

Yasmin and Yaz are contain ethinyl estradiol and drospirenone. The drospirenone makes this pill what is known as a potassium-sparing diuretic. As a diuretic Yasmin causes dehydration of a kind that affects the body at a cellular level and as such interferes with mineral and electrolyte balances. As a result potassium levels in the blood rise.

The effect on the body's potassium levels was addressed in the retraction commercial provided by Bayer at the FDA's insistence but as a stand-alone comment it is meaningless to most. Some of the effects of elevated potassium levels are nausea, fatigue, heart palpitations, numbness or tingling in limbs and muscle weakness. A serious impact is heart attack.

The diuretic action of these drugs prevents bloating and produces weight loss. However, the cellular dehydration that is a consequence has many negative effects on the whole body including increased allergies, irritable bowel syndrome, blood sugar imbalances, low energy, poor sleeping patterns, hair loss and pain from headaches to muscular aches. The dehydration also impacts on mood and triggers the "fight or flight" response. This response creates a constant stress on the body that inhibits digestion, raises stress hormones and increases blood pressure.

Yasmin and Yaz suppress adrenal gland function, as do all birth control pills, but as a potassium-sparing diuretic and anti-androgen they have other layers of impact on the body and mind.

The adrenal gland produces the stress-related hormones, one of which is cortisol. Suppression of the adrenal gland provokes a lowering of serum cortisol levels. Cortisol guides the body's responses to stress. Changed levels in serum cortisol are connected to depression and psychological stress. When the body experiences stress it provokes heightened adrenalin production. The long-term effect of high adrenalin levels is exhaustion. The adrenal glands also produce DHEA, which converts to testosterone, estrogen and progesterone when needed. The adrenal suppressing effect of the pill as a whole, but Yasmin and Yaz in particular, cause DHEA levels to drop, which in turn cause testosterone levels to drop dramatically. Testosterone plays a key role in libido in women as well as men and the capacity for mental and physical energy and is also converted to estrogen to help maintain bone density. Drospirenone has a particularly strong anti-androgen effect and wipes out testosterone.

The quashing of testosterone produces the skin-clearing effect of the drugs. Women's experiential statements suggest that Yaz and Yasmin potentially produce extreme mood changes and this anecdotal evidence corresponds with the known impact of cellular dehydration, elevated potassium, lowered testosterone levels, and suppression of the adrenal system. Adrenal fatigue is a health issue with a range of symptoms – fatigue, weakness, anxiety, depression, brain fog, and muscle pain. Alongside

Adrenal Fatigue, Flu Syndrome is mentioned in the insert as an extremely rare side effect.

The class action lawsuits against Bayer include users of drospirenone-containing drugs who have experienced blood clots, gallbladder disease, heart attack (myocardial infarcation), and stroke (cerebrovascular accident). For all the women who have experienced these serious physical side effects, there are many women who have experienced the relatively minor but still quality of life-threatening issues that are on the same spectrum.

The pill has an extensive, insidious effect on every bodily function.

The central impacts on the hormonal system and metabolic system have a build-up effect that changes women's mood and sense of well-being. The pill promotes vitamin deficiency as it prevents the body from properly and efficiently absorbing nutrients. Supplements are not helpful because they cannot be absorbed effectively by a metabolic system that is suppressed.

Sustaining the B vitamin complex including folic acid and iron and magnesium levels is particularly vital to maintaining neurological health and a balanced emotional state. The change in hormone levels impacts on the immune system function and disables its ability to protect the body from bacteria and allergens in the gut and the genitals.

The negative mood changes women experience can be traced back to changed hormone levels and fluctuations, vitamin deficiency, changes in glucose regulation, and changes in sodium and potassium levels.

On the pill no woman's body is capable of functioning at its optimum level. The body has a delicate system of balance and each woman's system is different, though every woman taking the pill will experience, over time, impaired physical and mental health.

In Susan Faludi's *Backlash* she writes, "The feminine woman is forever static and childlike...we see her silenced, infantilized and frozen." On the pill you are essentially "static." The suppression of ovulation and menstruation, indicators of entry into female adulthood, is physically infantilizing. When discussing side effects of the pill women often speak in terms that are illustrative of Faludi's description. They say they felt "trapped," "suppressed," "stultified," and "numb."

The pill's impact on the libido has been publicized but it is generally dismissed with humor. The libido is seen as distinct from women's emotional and physical health, whereas with men it is linked. The female sex drive is not celebrated or seen as essential to her femininity or sexuality. Women have been convinced that our desire for sex hinges on the psychological context whereas men's libido does not vary in accordance to their thoughts or feelings about circumstances. In lowering the hormone levels and flattening out the fluctuations the pill takes away the natural peak of libido women experience in connection with ovulation and sometimes pre-menstruation.

Research that indicates that lowered libido is experienced by a large number of women on the pill is undercut by the cultural assumption that most women have little real interest in sex regardless of this drug. Women joke with each other that this is how the pill actually works, via enforced abstinence.

One study suggested that for some women who take the pill their libido might never return to its pre-pill level, as the impact on testosterone levels is permanent.

Specifically the pill induces high levels of Sex Hormone Binding Globulin that bind to testosterone making it unusable and this effect often continues long after hormonal contraceptives are discontinued. This research is considered negligible and unimportant in the face of the presented benefits of the pill to women and, we assume, to men.

Nelly Oudshoorn in *Beyond the Natural Body* investigates how cultural notions of femaleness became part of the scientific understanding of women's bodies. "Scientists do not operate independently or outside of a social or political context. They actively select and create the contexts in which their claims may be made relevant," she writes. Through this merging of culture into medical practice we are led to believe the results are natural and inevitable.

As discussed, the ovaries were perceived as "organs of crises" from the nineteenth century. They became the pivotal point of the medical field of gynecology, which was invented in the late nineteenth century. An equivalent male reproductive science never came about, of course. It was in 1905 that hormones entered medical consciousness but it took two more decades before the pharmaceutical industry took control over the mass production of synthetic hormones for medical purposes. A major step in this process was the development of extraction techniques to remove hormones from inexpensive and available animal urine.

Although it was discovered that men have estrogens and progesterone in their bodies and women have testosterone, the hormones were divided up by those representing the newly created realm of sex endocrinology into female hormones and male hormones. It was decided by sex endocrinologists that women had a cyclical hormone regulation and men a "stable" hormone regulation. Today men are generally considered to have relatively stable hormone levels and women are described as having erratic and unpredictable hormone levels.

The male system is the norm and the female system is abnormal and so medicated to become more like the male model as it is perceived.

In their strong anti-androgen action Yaz and Yasmin are as such means for the ultra-feminization of the woman on a hormonal level. The "male" hormone of testosterone is wiped out leaving just the "female" hormones, albeit synthetic versions.

Oudshoorn asks how the discovery of hormones might have

developed if we lived in a culture that created an andrological clinic for men before the gynecological clinic for women?

The flipside of what happens to women's bodies when they are on the pill is what the hormone cycle and ovulation can do for us when they are not suppressed by drugs. As Laura Wershler, a veteran sexual and reproductive health advocate involved with Planned Parenthood associated organizations for over 25 years, states, "Let's not only think of what the pill does to a woman's body, but what her natural cycle could be doing for her."

...won't hurt you

So many women now only experience the fake period of the withdrawal bleed as a consequence of long-term use of the birth control pill from their teens onwards that it is just a small step to the situation we currently inhabit culturally in which not having a period at all is presented as preferential, both medically and socially.

At the release of the continuous oral contraceptive brands medical practitioners argued that because for much of history women had spent their fertile lives pregnant or breastfeeding menstruation is in fact biologically unnecessary and potentially dangerous. Their logic is that a functioning uterus and ovaries are more susceptible to going wrong than organs that are "switched off."

Within our culture in which periods are generally presented as disgusting and unfeminine women cannot have an opinion on their own periods that is free from this influence. Although some experience overbearing discomfort during menstruation, some do not and others feel the benefits of experiencing menstruation equal to or outweighing the cramps and inconvenience. Of course this culture plays its part in what women see as inconvenient and difficult. According to the medical industry we are all disabled by menstruation and the conversation is framed by this ideology.

There is no discussion of the benefit of ovulation. The emphasis on menstruation reveals the pervasive ignorance about women's biology, ignorance about the fact that menstruation and ovulation are paired phenomena. It also suggests a prevalent bias towards the elimination of periods. Those advocating for menstrual suppression claim that the pill kept women's reproductive organs "quiet and healthy."

Philosophy Professor Moira Howes in an article asked in response, "The quiescent uterus raises old value-laden associations between women and passivity. If the dormant, quiet, and weak uterus is healthy, is the active, energetic, and strong uterus unhealthy?"

Continuous or uninterrupted ovulation, that is ovulation not suppressed by drugs, is referred to by medical representatives as "incessant" – a term that carries negative connotations. Their thought is that working ovaries and a working uterus are subject to wear and tear much like a car engine. As Howes points out, this is not a line of thought attributed to the male production of sperm. In fact, here the opposite is true, an abundance of sperm production is linked to the perception of virility, strength and good health.

The acceptance of the myths surrounding menstruation is apolitical. The otherwise alternative thinking, progressive website *Alternet* published a piece titled 'Imagine Never Having to Have Your Period Again: The Truth About Menstruation.' Psychologist Valerie Tarico framed her argument for suppressing periods from a falsified status quo. To decide to stop having periods is described as a rebellion against the restrictive pressure put on women to have, and love, menstruation.

Tarico argues that women should be able to choose how often they have their period as though choosing the frequency with which their groceries are delivered. "Menstrual symptoms cause over 100 million lost hours of work for American women, they are the number one reason women miss school and work," she pronounces, adding that "there are no known long term consequences of menstrual suppression."

With echoes of the writings of Dalton from 1950 that reminded men of women's biological handicap, the article highlights that Italian research shows menstruation plays a significant part in maintaining the wage gap between men and women. It is, she argues, menstruation and not systematic misogyny and oppression that prevent women from earning the same as men for the same work. In the research documents we can see the researchers go to great pains to extrapolate from vastly generalized data that women may be taking more days off work than men due to menstruation. It is a presumptive and not proven observation. They may just as well be taking the time off to care for a sick child or relative, or catch up on the housework or because they're exhausted from doing all of the domestic duties that women generally take the most responsibility for on top of their office job.

We should, Tarico argues, be able to put personal choice for whatever reason above any cultural or social views on menstruation. She believes that menstruation holds a positive standing in present society and this prevents women from making their desired personal choice to "ditch" periods for good.

She describes menstruation as preventing women from succeeding in an array of arenas in life, "Some of us also like to dance in leotards, swim in bikinis, race in triathlons, work in military combat zones, backpack in bear country, or wear white in the summer."

This way of thinking emerges every few months in a spate of op-eds and news reports. It is given traction by Dr Elisimar M Coutinho's *Is Menstruation Obsolete?* Coutinho is an influential member of the World Health Organization. His research brought about the creation of the Depo Provera injection and implant, as well as other hormonal contraceptive methods. Coutinho's co-author on this book was Population Council Scientist Sheldon

Segal. With the perpetually pregnant cave woman as their standard for what is natural and good for women and their bodies, they argue for menstrual suppression via pharmaceutical drugs.

In an attempt to outwit any criticism in the preface it is written, "Some women have interpreted this book as an attack on menstruation and have resented the implication that there is something inherently wrong with the process." Ignoring much of history to create their own falsified narrative the writers set up their thesis to be a counter-attack to the prevalent belief that menstruation is "natural, normal and beneficial." They set themselves up as radical proponents of women's liberation from ignorance and primitivism, but they and their ideas are only products of a long history of misogyny-led medicine.

The perpetually pregnant cave woman is the ideal and they argue that women must return to this state albeit artificially through medication.

On this Dr Elizabeth Kissling writes, "Coutinho documents numerous menstrual maladies, such as premenstrual syndrome, anemia, endometriosis, dysmenorrhea, and menstrual migraine, combined with the anthropological inferences about the menstruation of our Paleolithic ancestors, and concludes "The attitude that menstruation is a 'natural event' and therefore beneficial to women in some way has no basis in scientific fact." Note also that Paleolithic women did not engage in such "unnatural" practices as shaving their legs, having their pubic hair removed with hot wax, or deliberately starving themselves to conform to an idealized body type. These practices all carry health risks, yet contemporary American women are widely encouraged to practice all three."

Although the female reproductive organs are considered to be only truly useful when in the process of creating a baby, pregnancy is problematic in the cultural narrative of hormonal contraceptives. Pregnancy is openly described in terms that suggest it to be a disease. It is said that there is a teen pregnancy "epidemic." The side effects of birth control pills are compared to that of pregnancy as though pregnancy were a sickness. In comparison to hormonal contraceptives the state is described as dangerous and risky, the most risky period in any woman's life. Yet, if you want to have a baby and choose to do so within a socially acceptable milieu and timeline then it becomes the best of female experiences.

The discussion of pregnancy as though it is a disease increases the fear surrounding fertility and restricts self-knowledge. We have been led to see a pregnant teenager as inherently wrong, no matter what the circumstances. The language used to discuss unwanted and wanted pregnancies is significantly contrasting and yet how do we decide what is an unwanted pregnancy and what is a "happy accident"? It is economic factors that bear most heavily on our conclusion.

In 2012 the pharmaceutical company Pfizer recalled one million packets of oral contraceptives due on a mix up in the sequencing of active and inactive pills it was asked in the media if the company would be liable for any unwanted pregnancies that occurred as a result of their mistake. The statement given by the company and medical practitioners was that women would not incur any "health risk," with no mention of pregnancy. Yet elsewhere we see pregnancy referred to as a greater "health risk" than birth control pills. The absence of an unwanted pregnancy is considered the most important, if not the only, sign of good health in young women.

Endocrinologist Dr Jerilynn Prior has studied menstruation and ovulation for over forty years. She is director of the Center for Menstrual Cycle Research (CeMCOR) at the University of British Columbia and has conducted research studies that suggest regular menstruation with consistent ovulation is the key to good heart, bone and breast health throughout a woman's life. She has produced protocols for alternative treatments for issues like heavy bleeding, irregular periods, period pain, endometriosis and PCOS for which the birth control pill alone is routinely prescribed. Dr Prior's provides strong evidence of the protective powers of ovulation for women's overall health.

"Ovulation and menstruation disturbances tell us the person is not healthy. Ovulation is the canary in the coal mine for women's health," Dr Prior states.

Sustaining ovulation through fertile years can help women avoid some of the major illnesses of our time like heart disease and breast cancer.

Although a woman may experience regular cycles she may not be ovulating, even when not on hormonal contraceptives. Addressing these ovulatory disturbances is the root of Dr Prior's work, and she feels, the root of preserving our health and longevity.

Research into women's cycles concentrates on menstruation and how often women experience their period. Dr Prior believes we should be looking at ovulation patterns also, as this can indicate and cause health issues. Ovulatory disturbances are what she terms the "silent" problem, invisible to the medical field. Irregular cycle lengths can be the last symptom of a health problem rather than the first.

A significant proportion of women not currently using hormonal contraceptives may not be ovulating regularly. A study conducted in Norway suggested as many as one third of women were not ovulating consistently.

Dr Prior finds it difficult to get the studies conducted at CeMCOR published with many rejected year after year for being "not interesting" or more suited to a "specialty" publication. As she says, "In Canada eighty-six percent of women will use the pill in their lifetimes – so what's specialty about this? The medical industry is authority-based and not science-based. They do not want to accept research that would change whole concepts."

A comprehensive study into bone density loss due to the pill was published only after three years of submissions.

Dr Prior states, "Most important is helping women to own their own cycles, that's that key to it. The feeling that men and women have, and they've probably never thought of it this way that their menstrual cycle belongs to a gynecologist or a GP or the pill is wrong. Your menstrual cycles, just like every other bit of you, like your elbow, like your foot, belong to you."

Although against the use of ovulation suppressing hormonal contraceptives, Dr Prior encourages women who want to use these drugs to keep a diary so that they can track the changes in their physical and emotional health it may cause. She sees diaries as an important tool in helping women find what is best for them. "The woman is her own best advocate," she believes.

Dr Prior presents the counter argument to the view of the medical establishment, the view we have all come to believe, that menstruation and ovulation are of no consequence beyond pregnancy and therefore hormonal birth control is safe and acceptable.

Through the CeMCOR website she provides treatment resources for healthcare providers and for women to pass on to their own doctors. Dr Prior wrote the book *The Estrogen Errors: Why Progesterone Is Better For Women's Health* and she prescribes a bio-identical progesterone, Prometrium, to women with ovulatory and menstrual issues.

Bio-identical hormones are still synthesized like non bio-identical hormones but are supposed to be more compatible with the body. However, they remain controversial in terms of their impact on the body and many people question whether they are really any improvement on non bio-identical synthetic hormones. Bio-identical progesterone creams are available over-the-counter, containing a significantly lower dosage of the hormone, and suggested for women going through menopause or suffering with PMS.

Although Dr Prior admits to CeMCOR receiving a one-off small donation for accommodations from the makers of Prometrium, Besins Health Care, she says she has never received payments or benefits from the company. Besins supplied, "at arm's length," the Prometrium used in studies into hot flushes in perimenopausal and menopausal women, but the Canadian Institutes for Health Research provided the funding.

In a piece for Bust magazine Rachel Friedman writes, "Like a person who endures the drawn out process of changing her diet and lifestyle instead of taking Lipitor at the first sign of high cholesterol, we too might want to consider non-pill treatment options. When it comes to a variety of women's health issues, we've basically got a one-pill-fits-all approach, and however each of us feels on and about the pill, we can all agree that that's unacceptable."

Clinical nutritionist Inna Topiler treats women with hormone imbalances. She believes, as Dr Prior argues, that excess estrogen as a result of hormonal contraceptives is a root of cancers, "I have had patients with breast cancer at an early age who were on the pill for a long time. I don't think the drug companies are making this connection publicly, but there are many people who are talking about it."

Excess estrogen can consequently lead to progesterone deficiency. Dr Prior's studies suggest progesterone to be an important factor in the maintenance of good health. Progesterone deficiency can impact on emotional and physical health and fertility.

Hormonal contraceptives are ranked by the World Health Organization as a class one carcinogen alongside tobacco and asbestos. They are believed to protect against the rarest form of female cancer, ovarian, which generally affects women over 70 years old. This benefit is frequently cited by medical professionals in the media. Pregnancy and breast-feeding also protect women from this cancer.

The protective effect of pregnancy on all forms of cancer is the presence of high levels of progesterone over an extended period of time, an effect that lasts for decades after the pregnancy. The protective effects by breastfeeding are the overall reduced levels of estrogen and progesterone when ovulation is suppressed.

The pill significantly increases women's risk of developing heart disease and breast, cervical and liver cancers. Recent research shows that if a woman starts taking the pill before she turns twenty her risk of developing breast cancer in later life is doubled. There are some that feel the pill should be considered on a par with the HPV virus as a co-carcinogen that can cause cervical cancer and ironically the immunosuppressant effect of the pill makes women more vulnerable to contracting HPV infections.

In recent years women who are perimenopausal and even post-menopausal have been encouraged to take the pill, with prominent media personality Dr Oz claiming women over forty should use it to cut the risk of ovarian cancer.

Alexandra Pope and Jane Bennett describe in *The Pill – Are You Sure It's For You* the non-lethal side effects of the pill as "quality of life-threatening." The health impact of the pill can be insidious and as such women will often put illnesses they experience down to the inevitable effect of growing older, stress or poor eating habits, without considering the root might be the pill.

The pill has been raised so high on its pedestal that the efficacy of all alternative contraceptive methods, including the barrier methods essential in reducing the transmission of STDs and HIV, have been undermined. Many women hold unrealistic evaluations of the pill's effectiveness as a result and they will cite perfect use instead of real life efficacy rates when speaking of the pill.

Condoms are victim to the dominance of hormonal contraceptives. Research has shown that a woman on the pill or another hormonal method is less likely to use condoms regularly in the early stages of a relationship. Condoms are viewed as messy and inconvenient in comparison.

In response to this anti-condom culture, in an article titled 'Love the Glove,' Heather Corrina writes, "If we're going to talk about condoms changing how sex feels, we need to remember that something like the pill does too, and unlike condoms, it changes how a woman feels all the time, both during and outside of sex. Condoms are the least intrusive and demanding of all methods of contraception. If guys could feel what life was like on the pill or get a Depo shot, they'd easily see condoms for the cakewalk they are."

Pill propaganda has eroded the fundamentals of reproductive rights – freedom, education and choice.

A woman who does not want to use the pill will have a hard time finding a doctor who will aid her with a diaphragm fitting and not hope to persuade her of its unsuitability as a contraceptive. She will only get to this point if she has been able to learn about the diaphragm and is not persuaded to switch brands of oral contraceptive instead or start on a different administration of hormonal birth control. Real choice and real freedom cannot be gained without comprehensive education.

When the pill was released women had to stand up to their doctors to get the pill, today they must fight to get off it.

Contemporary feminism is enamored with consumer choice and has fully accepted it as a substitute for freedom. When it comes to choosing a contraceptive method, it does not matter that women have not determined the range of choices. The experience that many women go through of swapping from brand to brand of hormonal contraceptive provides an illustration of freedom within the narrow range of choices.

Kissling writes on post-feminist media culture. She determines that post-feminism is performed by taking feminism into account only to dismiss it. Post-feminist media elevates above all the feminine body. It does not matter how a woman feels, only that she looks womanly.

Kissling examines the commercials for menstrual suppressant Seasonique, "The advert frames taking the pill as an act of defiance whilst incorporating key feminist values – self-definition, control of your body. The contradiction between controlling your body and submitting to the medical-industrial complex by taking the prescription is glossed over. They ask, 'Do you know there's no medical reason to have a period on the Pill?' They argue that it is not a real period, so there's no reason to have it. On Seasonique's website they call it a 'Pill period' and frame it in such a way to make it very easy to decide that having no periods is a good idea. The choice is that you're not menstruating or you are having a fake period - they don't compare Seasonique to the actual menstrual cycle. This normalizes being on hormonal contraception, as well as 'questioning' authority again - suggesting we are being duped into having periods we don't need."

Kissling argues that the non-menstruating female body fits well into the neo-liberal society. A non-menstruating body is always available, always "on" and it can therefore participate in the consumer economy continuously without a break. If we believe menstruation to be debilitating physically and mentally then we can believe that it must be suppressed in order to ensure women's full cooperation with the system.

Kissling states, "One member of the audience during my talk argued that it is 'more convenient' to not have periods. But it is inconvenient because of the way we define work in this economy."

There is a scene in the television show *Sex And The City* in which Charlotte, justifying her decision to Carrie to give up her job to be a housewife once she marries, agitatedly exclaims, "I choose my choice! I choose my choice!"

There are some, backed by the Society for Menstrual Cycle Research, who argues that menstruation is a sign of good health and should be treated as such. This was once standard medical practice, prior to hormonal contraceptives. Having periods is an indicator of healthiness on a par with blood pressure. In fact, a woman's cycle ensures her blood pressure is naturally lowered in the second half of the month. Monitoring teenagers and young women's cycles can ensure the early treatment of any arising health problems.

The Society for Menstrual Cycle Research presented a scientific forum to the New York Academy of Sciences proposing that the menstrual cycle be considered the fifth vital sign. "The menstrual cycle is a window into the general health and well-being of women, and not just a reproductive event," said Dr Paula Hillard at this event, professor of obstetrics & gynecology and pediatrics at the University of Cincinnati College of Medicine. "It can indicate the status of bone health, heart disease, and ovarian failure, as well as long-term fertility."

Teenagers who are not menstruating may be found to be suffering with an eating disorder, overwhelming stress, or physical issues such as polycystic ovaries, thyroid dysfunction or Cushing's disease.

It can take six years for the menstrual cycle to mature and the first three years are an adjustment phase that all women will go through. The teenage years are a time of bone growth. The pill promotes bone loss, which can lead to later-life osteoporosis. The hormonal injection Depo Provera, prescribed more so to teen girls than any other group, is particularly detrimental to bone health and warrants a black box warning in the insert.

During the maturation and adjustment phase teens are prescribed the pill and its derivatives. This is considered a medically based decision in the hands of GPs that has the added benefit of addressing pregnancy prevention. Normal issues that arise at this time are not treated but covered up by the drug even though there are effective treatments that truly bring about healthy, balanced cycles and alleviate the problems many teens experience like heavy bleeding and pain.

Dr Susan Rako writes in *No More Periods? The Risks of Menstrual Suppression* that we need to rework the discussion of hormonal contraceptives and acknowledge that drugs do not have "side effects," they only have "effects." Many of the major uses of top selling drugs were discovered first as "side effects."

An interesting comparison can be drawn with the campaign to claim sleep deprivation as a feminist issue. Arianna Huffington launched an initiative through *The Huffington Post* to encourage women to get eight hours of sleep at least regardless of their work or family duties. "Women have achieved so much already. Think what we can do if we're not tired!" she encouraged.

The issue is couched as such: women have sacrificed their natural, healthy sleep cycles in order to fit in with the demands of a heavily work-orientated society that demands long hours and increasingly levels of commitment to jobs. In order to achieve equal success and status in this society, women have been cutting back on their bedtime hours to the detriment of their health and their capacity for productivity. Huffington notes that disruption to the sleep cycle impacts on our flow of hormone levels and it is this that causes the resulting physical and mental health problems. Not getting enough sleep negatively impacts how our sex hormones function and it is this that causes the resulting physical and mental health problems and this not getting enough sleep over a long period of time can cause your body to work at a consistently less than optimal level.

The struggle to maintain a good sleep cycle against the social pressures to work late, rise early and maintain productivity holds parallels with the fight women must undertake when they choose to not use hormonal contraceptives against the pressures of the medical and pharmaceutical industries.

Huffington argues that if we were to leave our bodies to run through their health-ameliorating natural cycles at night and not tamper with this important element of our biology that women would achieve more, contribute more to society, and be more creative. As a result, she believes, society would benefit. Huffington does not just make the case based on a reader's need to feel refreshed in the morning, but extrapolates her thoughts to suggest a greater good could come from honoring this beneficial biological process. A process that has, in the same way as the monthly hormone cycle, been undermined and dismissed in deference to the structure of working life within our economy.

Women are encouraged to suppress their monthly ovulatory cycle in order to not miss any days of work or so as they can remain sexually available or experience only one-note moods.

Huffington can only see taking care of our bodies as a means to an end – becoming more productive, contributing more to the economy and acting as better members of that system. She does not consider that caring for our bodies might be a good idea even if it does not make us more productive. Our value as human beings, as women, is based on what we can produce.

We should be asking - what could women achieve if they weren't on the pill? What would women be if they weren't on the pill?

Keeping the secret

A pilot scheme began in London in 2009 to make the birth control pill available over-the-counter in areas of the city with the highest rates of teen pregnancy. In the aftermath of the US-based debate regarding access to birth control through health insurance many commentators asked if, seeing as the birth control pill is considered to be so safe, why is it not available without prescription? A *New York Times* writer argued that birth control pills are easy to use, require no need for instruction, safe and not addictive and so it would only make sense to have them available over-the-counter in pharmacies.

In 2012 when contraceptives were made "free" through health

insurance, the American College of OB/GYNs made the recommendation that birth control pills should be available without prescription. Their statement read, "Easier access to OCs should help lower the nation's high unintended pregnancy rate, a rate that has not changed over the past 20 years and costs taxpayers an estimated $11.1 billion annually. Cost, access, and convenience issues are common reasons why women do not use any form of contraception or use it inconsistently. There are no OCs currently approved for OTC access, but The College believes OTC availability will improve women's access to and usage of contraception. The benefits of making OCs easily accessible outweigh the risks."

There could be benefits from taking doctors out of the equation. Currently it seems as though few doctors provide sufficient and comprehensive healthcare to their pill-using patients. Serious physical side effects can be dismissed as unlikely, and quality of life-threatening effects can be dismissed as psychosomatic or put down to other issues.

Although this argument made by ACOG is indication of a widespread nonchalance and lack of knowledge about the pill's impact on the body, it is possible that fewer women would take the pill without the persuasive efforts of doctors. Fewer women might be persuaded to switch from one pill to another or from the pill to the injection or the patch with an assurance that the next option will have fewer side effects and make them feel better. They may decide to quit hormonal contraceptives earlier on and save themselves the side effects.

Women might be more likely to self-diagnose their own side effects and not rely solely on the wisdom of their practitioner. They might choose to stop taking hormonal contraceptives altogether if they are experiencing problems and have seen that other women have shared similar experiences online.

It seems, however, very doubtful that the pharmaceutical industry will give up their best-selling drugs to such a scheme when doctors are acting as their direct salesman. TV advertising is a part of the initial draw to a brand, but to persuade women to stay on the pill requires the hard sell of a trusted medical practitioner. Any drop in compliance as a result of cutting out the middlemen would equal a drop in profits.

It is important to the industry that the rejection of one pharmaceutical product provides an opening for the acceptance of another product, and not the rejection of all pharmaceutical options.

At the time of this announcement the promotion of so-called long acting reversible hormonal contraceptives reached new marketing heights with US state governments as well as the NHS running promotions to encourage women to learn more about these forms of contraception.

Dr. Susan E. Willis wrote on how the pharmaceutical industry backed President Obama's Affordable Care Act's provision for contraception because it eliminates a major barrier between women and these methods – cost: "Manufacturers of contraceptives have hundreds of millions of reasons to encourage the switch: their huge windfall from taxpayer-funded LARC will help offset the pharmaceuticals' settlements and liability judgments due to deaths and serious adverse events associated with the use of their products."

In the wake of the US LARC Awareness Week, in a piece for the Society for Menstrual Cycle Research, Wershler asked – "Do you love your LARC?" The California Family Health Council asked women to submit video testimonies explaining why they love their implant or IUD. Other LARCs such as the injection, patch and ring were not included in the campaign. Wershler highlighted stories online from women who had experienced serious side effects with these methods.

The 'Works Like A Charm' campaign from the National Campaign to Prevent Teen and Unplanned Pregnancy asked women to share stories about why they "love" their LARC in return for the chance to win $2,000 or an iPad. The website sported the line, "We love our LARCs because they let us get lucky without leaving anything to chance."

The implant and IUD are elevated above other methods because they ensure the highest level of compliance. A woman cannot independently stop using these contraceptives.

How likely is it in a culture of one-sided campaigns entitled 'Love My LARC' that doctors will take women's doubts and health concerns seriously?

The "myth busting" online events actually perpetuate misinformation and myths under the guise of truth telling in the face of misplaced anxiety. By merging the non-hormonal copper IUD and the hormonal IUD into the same group, the specific hormonal impact of the Mirena is ignored even though it has been shown to cause physical and emotional health problems.

The NHS has actively promoted long-acting hormonal methods of contraception for teens in a bid to lower the rate of teen pregnancy. For the NHS it is more cost-effective to provide long-term solutions that do not require consistent appointments with a health care provider or any follow up arrangements until the device is removed.

Planned Parenthood in the US has also put these methods at the forefront of their programs. Studies show that these methods have been pushed on the young and the poor in particular.

Currently in the US one in five African American teen girls are taking the injection. The rate of prescription reflects as nine percent of white teen girls to eighteen percent of black teen girls.

Lower income women who receive state-funded health care are more likely to be offered long-acting methods of contraception instead of the pill, particularly the shot or the implant. Long-term use of these methods, as with the pill, is critically under-researched. Depo Provera is currently also used in sex-offender rehabilitation programs to decrease sex drive.

Hormonal LARCs are presented as an improvement on the

pill. The articles that occasionally appear in women's magazines cautiously discussing the side effects of the pill experienced by so many of their readers suggest LARCs as the safe, modern alternative. Yet if a woman does experience negative changes in her body or mood whilst on a LARC she will have to wait some months before the problems will subside. A woman on the pill can choose to stop taking it from one day to the next without having to consult a doctor. Hormonal LARCs give yet more control to medical authorities and take what little power women have out of their hands.

As Wershler writes, "Throughout the contraceptive realm, LARCs are being heralded as the best thing since Cinderella's glass slipper with little acknowledgement that for many women LARCs are more like Snow White's poisoned apple."

Section Three: The Hook

"When the history of the 20th century is written, it may be seen as the first when men and women were truly partners. Wonderful things can come in small packages." The Economist names the birth control pill one of the Seven Wonders of the Modern World.

"I began Yaz to treat moderate acne. It's helped to dramatically clear my skin, but I've been having mood swings that range from absolute fury to mild irritation to deep sadness but I am rarely ever very happy any longer. I hope that will improve soon, because it's doing such a bang-up job on my skin and has increased my breast size." – Sara

Safe, effective, easy

The "safe, effective, easy" mantra is reiterated at the release of every piece of new research about the impact of the pill on the body and in response to women voicing their doubts. Women believe that the lower the dose of hormones in the brand of pill prescribed the safer the drug.

The idea that lower hormone levels equal a safer pill arises from the controversy that surrounded the original pill brands, which had a high level of synthetic estrogen. As new pills are released women understand them to be improved versions, just as a new form of laundry soap would be understood to be a better version of the previously available product. The pill is cited as being "safe," "safer than aspirin" is the frequently used analogy, because it has been available for decades. Yet over those decades many variations have evolved. Different brands of pill are the same in many ways and yet they are different in some important elements. Yasmin and Yaz are amongst the latest versions of the pill and said to be "low hormone."

As women take these drugs for longer and longer periods of their fertile life they are being drawn into an experiment group on which to test each new brand and the real long-term impact of the previous brands. The only desired outcome of this experiment is less unwanted pregnancies. A successful test therefore will see more women taking hormonal contraceptives than before. The health impact is not a factor for consideration.

Taking the pill in practice is not as effective as women are led to believe. When a woman does not know how this drug works to control her fertility or therefore how her body works she might be more inclined to take the tablets more casually than is needed for them to be fully effective. The connection between the method and its means is severed and as such there are missed pills and late pills and unwanted pregnancies.

In the US pill packets come with up to a week's worth of sugar pills for the monthly fake period break. The reasoning behind this is that as long as women keep up the ritual of taking a tablet every day they won't miss any once the medical cycle starts again. Even though intellectually women know that the sugar pills are useless most will take them in habit rather than throw them out. The cultural presentation of the pill as harmless encourages the blurring of the line between the placebo and the pill and allows women to unconsciously, unthinkingly continue to choose this form of contraceptive for their bodies every day.

Dr Claudia Panzer, a research scientist who conducted an important study regarding the pill's impact on free testosterone levels, remarked in the media that the pill is "handed out like candy."

In 2011 a brand of oral contraceptive was released called FemCon Fe that differentiated itself in the saturated market by its spearmint flavor. Women were able to chew the pill rather than just swallow, as though it were breath-freshening gum. It was marketed as convenient, even more so than all the other pills that might require a glass of water to be taken, and tasty.

Science is equated with progress, criticism of science as anti-progress. Women see themselves as protected by science from the suffering they have been told is God's will for their sex or "Eve's curse" as it is sometimes called. In the documentary *The Business of Being Born* it is highlighted that women gratefully took up the pain-relieving drugs used for labor pains that were provided by the medical establishment. Women's liberation activists hailed these new scientific inventions as an indication of the support for women's equal standing in society. The drugs were a dismissal of the justification for sexism established in the concept of Eve's curse. Women were happy to be sedated during labor then just as now many women are happy to have an epidural.

The documentary explores how the US has astonishingly high infant mortality and maternal mortality rates for a rich, western country. Women have been encouraged to be scared and suspicious of alternatives to the medical industry's sanctioned way of processing women through labor. Parallels could be drawn with how women are led to believe that alternatives to hormonal contraceptives are ineffective or unsafe. Pregnant women are told that an epidural and a cesarean are the best options available to them and the safest for themselves and the baby. This surgery-based system of labor and birth serves the medical industry in that it is relatively quickly and easily implemented by surgeons and provides a rapid and predictable turnaround time. It is, essentially, the most profitable system. A natural birth can go on for hours, days even. However, as evidenced in the mortality rates, this is for the many women who would go through a typical natural birth with few or no complications, not in their best interest or the best interest of their child.

Both women who turn down the standard hospital birth and those who decline hormonal contraceptives are considered selfish or deluded.

In both contraceptive and birth choices the medical industry actively discourages choice at the expense of women's health for the profit of the system.

Producer Ricki Lake has described the catalyst for her involvement in this on-going project as her "empowering" and "life-changing" choice to have a home birth. Women describe the experience of coming off hormonal contraceptives after a number of years in the same way.

There are profound similarities between the medicalization of birth and the medical control of contraception. For both areas this is justified under the banner of "safe, effective, easy" – the means justifies the end. Women do not choose an epidural or choose hormonal contraceptives because these things are necessary or convenient for them or because they consciously need or want to. They choose these things because they are ingrained as the 'right' choice to the point that it becomes the only choice.

Women are detached from the experience of a natural birth and from their experience of a natural hormone cycle through systematic medical intervention. The rapidly rising rate of cesarean sections is comparative to the rising prescriptions of long acting hormonal methods of contraception. Both may save money, time and are more convenient to hospitals, doctors and insurance companies but they hold massive drawbacks to health and well-being.

Neither pregnancy nor fertility should be viewed as an illness that requires treatment with pharmaceuticals or surgery.

The director of the documentary, Abbie Epstein, speaks to this one-size-fits-all attitude towards women's bodies when she writes, "In a culture where all our rituals have become standardized and commercialized, birth is the one rite of passage that can remain individualized and sacred if parents are exposed to the truth behind the medical myths."

Scientists can be used as apologists for the status quo. Scientific researchers only find what they start out looking for, especially when they are funded by the pharmaceutical industry.

Today's generation of women live in a technocratic society and respect that. They too will believe scientific discoveries that lead to development of technologies to be the only cure for all the world's ills, whether they are personal or global. Yet the scientists enacting science are impacted by their culture and are not free from its beliefs and prejudices. Science has long been used to justify the oppression of women and perhaps it is ignorance of this history that causes women to so enthusiastically and unquestioningly accept drugs and devices as their liberators.

The drug JQ1, currently in the animal testing stages, could prohibit sperm production without impacting men's hormone levels. In an article regarding this developing method Diana Blithe, program director for contraceptive development at the U.S. National Institute of Child Health and Human Development remarked to the media that the hormone-based drugs for men that are also under research are unlikely to reach the market as they block testosterone production and "inhibit the whole cycle."

Attention has been turned to non-hormonal contraceptives for men to avoid the problems associated with suppressing their natural hormone production.

Blithe advised that men temper their excitement for a new male-centered contraceptive with caution, "It's going to be many years before we see anything that could approach a product on the market because the level of safety for developing a contraceptive is very, very high. You're giving it to healthy people for a very long period of time so you have to have a product that's very effective and not going to cause side effects."

Also under research is a gel contraceptive that would physically block sperm and an ultrasound device to incapacitate sperm. Potential hormonal contraceptives for men have frequently come up against criticism for their high level of "unacceptable" side effects.

In 2011 a large study of a hormonal contraceptive for men was called off due to "higher than expected rates of minor side effects such as irritability and acne."

In a BBC documentary about our relationship to the long-term medications that we take, research scientists working on a hormonal contraceptive for men were asked what they saw for the future of such a drug. One researcher responds with an explanation of the acceptability issues surrounding stopping sperm production. It is, he described, like "tinkering at the heart of what makes a man a man." The researcher argues that if the female birth control pill were first introduced today it would not be welcomed.

The documentary narrator summarizes the conversation with, "A man without sperm. No more radical than what millions of women endure."

The documentary concludes with an ominous prediction for the future of the pharmaceutical industry: "A drug company's dream would be a pill not designed for sick people, but for everyone. A pill that's not good for you, but good for everybody and you are part of everybody." The future would be drugs that address risk factors rather than illnesses. The birth control pill treats the risk factor of pregnancy. The pill is promoted as good for every woman's body from teens through to the post-menopausal.

As population control is good for the health of a whole society, so the pill is good for everyone and women are part of everyone. We are already experiencing this feared future.

The greater good

The pill has what Barbara Seaman described as "diplomatic immunity" because its continued use is seen as a social good. Contraceptive culture in the US and UK is driven by the implementation of methods on the populations of developing countries. Population control underlines much of the conversation within the medical field about hormonal contraceptives.

The prevention of unwanted pregnancy is the overarching motivation and the only guiding force of those involved in providing contraceptive choices to women at home and abroad.

Although women in the US and UK are in a very different situation to those in developing countries, even if they are part of the astonishing number living below the poverty line, the way they are treated is very similar to those women in the third world when it comes to contraception.

Betsy Hartmann argues in *Reproductive Rights and Wrongs* that overpopulation is not the root cause of poverty. Contraceptive programs everywhere are dominated by a drive to reduce birth rates regardless of the consequences. The health and safety of women does not come into the planning or implementation. When concerns are raised they are quickly dismissed as unimportant when compared to the goal of preventing poverty through population control. It is thought that if women are prevented from having babies then their life conditions will improve, as will the conditions of their country.

Hartmann believes that the most effective and conscientious way to reduce the birth rate in a developing country would be to challenge its system of patriarchal power. She believes women should be provided with support, opportunities to learn, options to earn money, and provided with decision-making power over their lives. This alone she says will stabilize an economy. Instead crusading on limiting the number of children impoverished women birth by any means possible, regardless of the consequences to their health, is neither compassionate nor effective in the long-term. It is a logic founded in a patriarchal ideology that purposefully and willfully ignores the real source of inequality.

In the US and UK advocates for hormonal contraceptives will often refer to population control to provide power to their arguments. They are happy to see poverty as a simple equation of too many people and too few resources and even happier to be prescriptive about how women in developing countries should be recruited to fix this problem. The same logic is applied to the contraception discussion within their own countries. We must not openly discuss health and safety issues as instilling these doubts in the most used contraceptives inevitably raises the number of unwanted pregnancies.

That even liberal feminists use this argument as though it were an undeniable truth reveals the insidiousness of the pill myth. They do not consider it necessary to better the power relations between men and women in those countries, nor to support women in their desire to gain equality. When the pill was released the male to female relationships were very different to what they are today, yet we have not seen a reassessment of contraception in view of this change. Society demands that women must be sexually available. Feminists assume women have to be sexually available. The idea that women can't, won't or don't say no to sex underlies the belief system that perpetuates pill use.

The pill is a hidden, invisible and non-disruptive method. At that time of the pill's release it was thought to be better to medicate women and make contraception their sole responsibility than to consider the possibility that men and women could be equal partners in a conversation about birth control.

Hartmann outlines that if there is a high infant mortality rate in a country then the women will have more children in the knowledge that many will die before they become adults. Women living in poverty need children in order to survive. Children can help them with work, and can take care of them as they get older or become ill. The assumption is that women do not want or need many children and that they are always unwillingly pregnant.

Many of the women in developing countries who are prescribed hormonal contraceptives experience side effects and will stop taking them. Those in developing countries are unlikely to return to the doctor once this happens. If one woman has unwanted side effects she will tell other women and they will be warned off working with the visiting doctors. Women in developing countries are told even less than we are in developed countries about the potential pitfalls of hormonal methods or the symptoms to watch for if side effects are taking hold.

If a woman has low body weight, poor nutrition and lives in circumstances with poor sanitation putting her on hormonal contraceptives with no health screening could cause serious health problems that outstrip those we see in the western world. These methods prevent the absorption of vitamins and negatively impact the functioning of metabolic system as a whole and so can cause women to become further malnourished and weakened.

A women already struggling with poor health will find she becomes sick more often and for longer periods when using hormonal contraceptives because her body is not working at optimum level, from the immune system through to blood sugar balance.

Some long-acting hormonal methods like the injection can cause continuous bleeding – even though they're advertised as having the benefit of stopping periods altogether – and women in developing countries often cannot afford to lose the blood and the iron it contains at such a rate. With limited access to sanitary products and sanitation in general this can be a source of stress and sickness. They will also be, where menstrual taboos are strictly enforced, ostracized socially for the continuous bleeding.

Long acting methods, especially the implant and the injection, are popular in developing nations because they are cheaper and increase compliance. A woman provided with a packet of pills may stop taking them. The dominance of hormonal methods of contraception worldwide discourages research into other non-hormonal methods. Although it is barrier methods that greatly reduce the spread of STDs and HIV they are not at the forefront of many contraceptive programs.

In 2011 the New York Times published a front-page article on research that claimed the hormonal contraceptive injection Depo Provera doubles the risk of transmission and acquisition of HIV. The largest study of its kind conducted by Renee Heffron in Africa found that HIV-negative women being given the shot every three months had twice the risk of contracting the virus and that HIV-positive women were twice as likely to pass the virus on to their partners.

In 2012 the World Health Organization made a statement that the research was not broad or deep enough to be conclusive and recommended Depo Provera continue to be administered with no restrictions in addition to encouragement of the use of condoms. In response the headlines of national newspapers reported falsely that there was no concern of a link between the method and HIV.

Currently in Sub-Saharan Africa where HIV is most rampant the contraceptive injection is the most widely used method of birth control, with 12 million women on Depo and oral contraceptives used by 11 million. The contraceptives' effectiveness, invisibility, lack of daily routine and its requirement of only four visits to a medical professional per year have made it the most widely distributed birth control method in that area.

In 2012 the Bill and Melinda Gates Foundation presented its strategy to get the Depo Provera shot to millions more women in Africa and South Asia. In her recent TED talk Melinda Gates discussed how "popular" the injection is with African women. The Gates Foundation is partnered with the pharmaceutical company Pfizer – the maker of Depo Provera – in this mission. The company has produced Uniject, which is a shot that can go under the skin instead of intramuscularly and so does not require a doctor for its use and can be administered by the woman herself. Billions of dollars have been poured into increasing uptake of this particular method in developing countries.

Hartmann wrote in response, "For over a decade now studies have pointed to a possible link between Depo Provera use and increased risk of acquiring HIV...Precaution would dictate that

Depo be phased out in populations at high risk of AIDS, but instead the WHO has thrown caution to the wind...At a time when Depo Provera should be under intense scrutiny, the Gates initiative is vigorously promoting it, along with a Chinese hormonal implant, as the two main contraceptive technical fixes for sub-Saharan Africa and South Asia."

Hartmann has reported on the incentives received by clinics in Africa that provide the most women with the recommended forms of birth control. There have been reports of direct coercion of women via bribes and threats. "It's shocking how little critical concern there is, especially amongst women's health activists," said Hartmann. "Unfortunately the vacuum is being filled by anti-abortion groups who are taking on the role of investigators highlighting the problems with Depo."

There is no evidence to show that population density causes lack of resources and poverty although this is the message the Gates Foundation works under, that decreasing birth rates will elevate the economic status of countries and promote development. Hartmann points out that multi-national corporations that own much land in developing countries push populations into unsuitable areas for farming and living in order to take advantage of better areas and this oppression from the outside as well as the linked corruption of the governments are key causes of continued poor living conditions for many Africans.

Hartmann calls population control a "substitute" for social justice that holds back the emancipation of women.

She asserts that real reproductive choice relies on women having control over their own lives and equal power to men and this can only come with economic development. Developed nations are uninterested in providing aid for such countries, because they are active in their exploitation via cooperation with corrupt governments and via the corporate power wielded over those countries. The people are purposely kept poor so that developed countries (or at least their corporations) can become richer.

Melinda Gates has taken up contraception as her own personal crusade. In reaction to US debate and on-going cultural control of the religious Right, she has said that contraception should not be seen as a "controversial" issue. The answer to poverty, as she sees it, is increased funding for more hormonal contraceptives and creating better access in developing countries. "One of the simplest and most transformative things we can do is give people access to birth control," she states.

Gates admits that other issues of inequality should be addressed but, she believes, these may be far too complex and too political to be considered. Drawing from her Catholic background she believes that religious conservativism rules the conversation. She is correct in that the religious Right took hold of politics during the Reagan presidency and by linking abortion and contraception prevented funding for research.

The population control crusade to distribute the most effective form of contraception and not the best for women's health and situation is rooted in fundamental anti-female ideology.

Pregnancy is made to be the problem and not the poverty itself. This belief is reflected in developed nations where we see that unwanted pregnancy is framed as the worst possible event in a woman's life, centrally because it will prevent her personal progression through the accepted timeline that allows for a succession of school, college, work, money, career, relationship, babies - in that order. A step outside of that structure is unsupported culturally and financially.

The US or UK teen pregnancy epidemic as is not treated with education but medication. Pregnancy is the cause of destitution in this narrative, not the reverse. If pregnancy outside of the prescribed timeline does indeed cause destitution that is not the fault of the woman with the unwanted pregnancy but the fault of a society that discourages education and denies her financial and social support. If a teenager has a child at seventeen she should still have the option of going to college or getting a job, the only reason she is isolated is because our society wills it that way.

Bitch magazine writer Katherine Don investigates the pregnancy as disease and teen pregnancy as epidemic equation, "All told, the disease framework legitimizes intolerance against pregnant women and moms. Why demand choice when you didn't sufficiently "protect yourself"? Why institute paid parental leave when mom unnecessarily allowed herself to contract pregnancy? Why demand economic justice when you're the one who got yourself "into this mess"? Why require that dad pay child support when it's mom who didn't prevent her "condition"? In a healthcare system that treats even a socially sanctioned pregnancy as a "burden to the system," every woman is part of an "at-risk" population, and every pregnancy is conceived of as a disease."

Population control was, of course, the argument wielded by Margaret Sanger in her fight to provide effective contraception for women. Sanger rationalized the need for access to contraception and the need for the development of an oral contraceptive by describing a need for population control amongst the poor of the United States. This argument appealed to those from whom she needed support much more so than any avocation for women's rights could.

Although involved in the feminist and socialist beginnings of the work for contraceptive choice and access, she came up against strong opposition from the male dominated governmental bodies and changed her presentation of the argument drastically in response. The thought that society could prevent the "wrong" people from having children was appealing to those she required on her side for the success of her plans.

In her work Susan Rako calls attention to the Hippocratic Oath – "Above all, do no harm" - and its promise to put the interests of the individual before those of the society.

Elaine Tyler May writes in *America and the Pill* that in the

1950s and 1960s, "Many saw the pill as a "magic bullet" that would avert the explosion of a "population bomb." By reducing the population it would alleviate the conditions of poverty and unrest that might lead developing nations to embrace communism. Population control, it was believed, would promote growth of markets for consumer goods and the emergence of capitalism.

The pill was to be "the key to social order" and "a means to an end with success marked by the achievement of national and global transformation."

We see evidence of this theory in the contemporary approach to contraception. The governments of developed countries are reluctant to provide aid to developing countries that might, in elevating their living conditions, bring about rebellion against the multi-national corporations that have a stronghold over their land, resources and communities. Even, or perhaps especially, a comparatively generous billionaire like Gates cannot fathom an alternative to the current situation for the poverty-stricken. She views the issues facing them other than simple family size as too complex for her or us to understand or even begin to tackle. Gates' attitude is as paternalistic as the supporters Sanger sought.

Gates believes herself to be a compassionate liberal. She says - If only there were less poor, they would be easy to deal with. Fewer children in poverty would be less of a burden on the conscience. To raise the issue that rich countries consume too much at the expense of others would be to admit fault with the system that provides for the few and open up the possibility that there might be another, perhaps better way. Gates has benefitted so well from the capitalist system she does not have the capacity to criticize.

Barbara Seaman believed the population control argument to be a "panacea" just as the pill is a "panacea" for the "problem" of being female in a male dominated and defined society.

Sealing the deal

Faced with fanaticism on both sides – the religious conservatives of America wanting to see a ban on all contraceptives and the liberal Democrats wanting to see every woman on long acting hormonal contraceptives – it's no wonder that women became defensive of their freedom of contraceptive choice.

Upon hearing the news that insurance companies under the Affordable Care Act would have to provide contraceptives 'free' of charge, women joked openly that they would be gorging, overdosing, greedily gulping down birth control pills from now on.

In an interview reported under the headline, 'Katy Perry Pops Birth Control Like Skittles' the pop star said, "I basically chew my birth control tablets – I chew them like vitamin C, I'm like 'nomnomnomnom.'"

Far right conservative Rush Limbaugh remarked on his radio show that a young woman who was making the case for birth control coverage to the House of Representatives was a slut for wanting to have the pill "for free." His remark, however misogynistic, did raise questions that the debate had otherwise let alone. Why do women take a pill every day to prevent pregnancy? If they are taking a medication every day to have sex without the risk of pregnancy, Rush Limbaugh's logic summarized, they must be having a lot of sex.

It was the skewed conclusion of an inflammatory provocateur but it pushed those pro-access to argue that the pill is used for many reasons other than pregnancy prevention, including medical conditions like endometriosis and PCOS. In the UK if you are using the pill for contraception, you receive it for free. If you are using it for acne, you have to pay the nominal sum for the prescription. Yet the UK is not burdened with the moralistic posturing and pseudo-religious justification that is used in the US to stir up the social conservatives. States looked to legislate bills that allow employers providing health insurance to mandate whether their employee was using the birth control for the morally right reason, for a medical issue.

Actress Elizabeth Banks was recruited during by Planned Parenthood to create a video in which she would admit to using "birth control" – as discussed a term used interchangeably with hormonal contraceptives and generally not in reference to any other form of contraception – for migraine headaches and a "heavy flow." The pro-access told the religious Right what it wanted, or needed, to hear. It was a reflection of the early years of Margaret Sanger's fight when she argued for pregnancy to be defined as a disease so that she could gain support for a contraceptive drug as its "treatment."

The contemporary argument was taken back in time and the birth control pill repositioned as a radical device encouraging and enabling rebellion against oppressive forces.

When women share their experience of side effects online, Kissling has noted that women are more likely to blame themselves for a lack of proactive, engaged choice-making and insufficient self-monitoring than any of the systematic issues of advertising, corrupt relations between doctors and pharmaceutical companies or the for-profit healthcare system. That their contraceptive choice caused them to become depressed, paranoid or agoraphobic, break up with their boyfriend or lose their job is, as they see it, no one's fault but their own. They berate themselves for not taking notice of the package inserts, not questioning their doctor and then for having a faulty body that does not "accept" these synthetic hormones quietly.

Kissling argues in her essay 'What does not kill you makes you stronger' that the neo-liberal woman will view any notion that undermines her agency and freedom as a conspiracy theory. She will not doubt her own freedom from external pressures. She is self-actualizing and as a consumer wields the ultimate power. Her inability to correctly choose the right hormonal contraceptive for her body is viewed with a disdain for her aptitude as a consumer. Their reactions to the experience of side effects are the result of making choices under the illusion of freedom. A neoliberal will turn against and scold her body for non-compliance to the drugs.

Kissling argues that, "The non-menstruating woman is the ideal neoliberal subject. A women's menstruating body is leaky, it swells, it's unpredictable, her emotions are heightened – therefore this body is seen as a problem in a neoliberal economy. A menstruating woman can't present herself as a rational, self-actualizing subject; she isn't able to participate in consumerism 24/7. A non-menstruating body is much better suited to market success in the consumer economy."

Wendy Brown provides foundation for this view, "Neo-liberalism normatively constructs and interpolates individuals as rational, calculating creatures whose moral autonomy is measured by their capacity for 'self-care' – their ability to provide for their own needs and serve their own ambitions. The capitalist free-market rules all. It is necessary that women are fully available, including sexually available."

Kissling highlights that she sees no sense of any need for women to take collective action in response to the issues they are experiencing with these drugs, even when those issues mount up and correlate and even as it becomes undeniable that these problems are caused by the drugs and impact a vast number of women. They will share their stories and support each other with tips and advice but it is down to the individual to change her own personal situation. The first available and widely known collective act might be to report the side effects to the FDA. Women cannot be blamed for feeling that this would be futile in view of the regulatory body's conduct in the case of Yaz and Yasmin. It is not likely many women have heard of this case, therefore their disinterest in this option reveals a sense of isolation.

Natasha Walter and Ariel Levy in their respective books *Living Dolls* and *Female Chauvinist Pigs* argue that sexual agency has become a substitute for real freedom. When this is coupled with the freedom of consumer choice we have a situation is which being able to have sex when you want, with who you want, as much as you want and however you want is the ultimate badge of empowerment and liberation. The pill and now more so the convenience and forgettable nature of the patch, shot, ring, IUD or implant are seen as facilitators of this freedom. If these facilitators cause health issues women do not consider themselves duped.

The faith in the free market as a cure-all in itself prevents us from seeing that we are not taking control of our bodies so much as being controlled.

Section Four: The Addict

"Because her body is suspect to her, and because she views it with alarm, it seems to her to be sick, it is sick." Simone De Beauvoir, *The Second Sex*

"I went on Yaz to control my bleeding. I got off it five months ago only to return to it one cycle later. I noticed the difference quickly, when I stopped I felt clearer. I didn't realize I had brain fog until then. But I was bloated and breaking out, I missed the diuretic and the clear skin. I am so mad with myself because I am thinking I should get off it again. I could continue being anxious and weak and wondering if I am getting sick or I can try again. I'm so scared to go through the up and down again. It's like an addicting drug. I have been having sharp pain in my chest. I can always feel my heart beating fast and loud. I have very little interest in a social life. Hoping to quit next month." – Heidi

Muted

The pill promotes and perpetuates women's trained suspicion and distrust of their own bodies and biology.

Wolf writes that the economy requires "passivity, anxiety and emotionality." These attributes are supported by the widespread use of hormonal contraceptives. Wolf argues that women are required to be both "sexually available and sexually insecure." Through the combination of lowering libido, suppressing physically heightened sexuality by preventing ovulation and producing depressive symptoms hormonal contraceptives hold women in a state of sexual insecurity. Women on the pill describe feeling detached from reality, numbed, foggy headed, and as though living "behind a veil." The more anxious, self-doubting, and fearful a woman feels the more she will want to shop to feel bolstered and better. It is comforting, soothing to buy when you need to believe a purchase might make your life better.

Wolf concludes that society has no interest in the health or appearance of women, only in keeping women happy to be told what they can and cannot do.

Tyler May reports on the support Hugh Hefner gave for the pill. The Playboy brand founder determined that the pill would allow for "uninhibited sex" and therefore would make women more open to sex, more interested in sex and, he hoped, more openly sexy.

Hefner voiced his belief that women who did not want to take the pill were "neurotic, prudish and hostile to men." In the pages of Playboy magazine he wrote that women should happily tolerate any side effects and embrace instead the benefits the pill provides to their "sexuality."

Hefner's marker of improved sexuality was an increase in the amount of sex a woman had with her partner. He did not consider women's sexuality to exist outside of its relation to sex. Although men have a continuous sense of masculinity, women do are not thought to need a sense of femaleness any more complicated than a physical performed sexiness that is attractive to men. Hefner decided that if a woman looks sexy and is having sex then she must be experiencing a liberated sexuality.

Women today are asked to believe that as long as they look outwardly appropriately feminine that they should not be concerned with what is going on inside their bodies.

Women complain that the men in influential and powerful positions do not understand their bodies. The string of Republican representatives making outlandish claims about women's reproductive biology rightfully incite horror amongst women's health activists. However, the truth is that very few of these women have an understanding of their bodies themselves.

It is during surges of protest against the oppression of women's reproductive rights that lack of education becomes the most apparent. Those women who take a keen interest in their diets, their exercise regime and their fitness, those otherwise most in touch with their physical self, have a blind spot when it comes to hormonal contraceptives.

The pill is believed to be a help and not a hindrance to good health. Good health translates for women as perfect appearance. External signs of good health are traded off for the benefits of actual optimal physical and mental health.

The terror of pregnancy is connected to the shame of menstruation and together they provoke what Wolf termed "dread of lost control." Women's enthusiasm for hormonal contraceptives is anchored by this dread. An un-medicated female body is a dangerous, unpredictable and difficult body. Yet even as women experience the emotional and physical side effects of hormonal contraceptives they see this as their only option. Stopping and returning to a sense of lost control is too frightening a choice.

As Tony Benn remarks in Michael Moore's documentary *Sicko*, "An educated, healthy and confident nation is harder to govern," echoing Wolf's theory on the facilitation of women's oppression.

When women choose to come off hormonal contraceptives in order to get pregnant they find that they do not know how long it might take for the synthetic hormones to leave their body, when they might expect the return of their menstrual cycle or when they are fertile. Most expect to immediately return to regular cycles with ovulation. They also assume that the problems they had with their cycles before going on the pill have been treated and resolved by the drug.

The industry that has grown up around infertility issues is fed by this ignorance.

Women ask for and are offered IVF options within a shorter period of time than is realistic for achieving a pregnancy. They'll ask for infertility treatment before it should be certain that they need it because they are unaware that their body could take a year to readjust to its natural cycle. Few women know that they could aid the process by tracking their ovulation carefully and effectively. Many rely on expensive ovulation testing kits that may provide incorrect information or are useless without additional awareness of the cycle. They are often told there is a time when they are "most" fertile rather than that there are times when they are not fertile at all. If you are having sex every day of the month without realizing the majority of those days you are infertile the disappointment must be magnified.

Women are labeled infertile when they are in fact in recovery from hormonal contraceptives. They are not offered any treatments to return them to healthy, ovulatory cycles that would restore their fertility. The medical industry combined with the pharmaceutical industry continues to exert power by capitalizing on this disconnect.

A research study polled women seeking fertility assistance at clinics. Only thirteen percent of women could correctly answer the question of when they were fertile in their cycle, although sixty-eight percent claimed they were already timing sex to their fertile period in the hope of getting pregnant. The lead researcher, Kerry Hampton, said that she felt this lack of awareness was contributing to the ever-increasing infertility "problem."

Tyler May quotes a woman as stating, "The pill helped me own my identity as a woman and be in control of my life, my body and my future." In contrast to this thought, Dr Prior suggests, "There's an emotional identity attached to achieving your own menstrual cycle, and being able to read your body. When you're on the pill, it's the doctor who's controlling your cycle. You don't own it."

It seems unlikely that May's interviewee would discuss a different drug in such dramatic, conceptual terms, not an asthma inhaler or an insulin injection, although they might have tangible life-saving purpose. This is a grand description for a drug that we are told deserves no scrutiny or serious consideration.

During the debate over implementing Affordable Care Act a commenter on a Huffington Post article remarked that if oral contraceptives could be made 'free' through health insurance then men should also be able to get their vitamins and supplements for free. These prevent illness just as the pill prevents the illness of pregnancy. We are told the pill is something close to an immunization against uterine and ovarian cancer. We are told it is protecting us from the health hazard of menstruation. The pill, like vitamins, we understand to have no detrimental effects on the body.

So it is remarkable that a woman would associate the pill with the formation of her identity. If she didn't own her body before taking the pill, who did?

We could agree that the identity the woman refers to is the social concept of femaleness and it is an image that women can only get close to through taking the pill. The history of femaleness has marked the present day identity of women. The phrase "taking ownership" sounds rebellious but could mean the woman is choosing to commit fully to the identity she knows, that social presentation of what it is to be a woman. The pill is there to help if you don't feel, look or behave the way society tells you that you ought in order to be an authentic, acceptable, real woman.

The woman chooses to take the pill to fit and make her way through society with less anxiety about not belonging.

May quotes another woman as saying that her choice to take oral contraceptives is "a non-issue – like brushing my teeth." Teeth brushing is something we are taught to do before we even know why it is that we should be doing it or what consequence it has to our body and our life experience. Teeth brushing is a ritual before it is a conscious action and so it would seem is taking the pill.

May also quotes this woman – "I just couldn't picture a fully-functioning society without the Pill, it's like asking what the impact of the telephone is." By that logic questioning the pill is inextricably linked to questioning present social structures.

Feminist writer Laurie Penny posted a photo of herself on her blog in which she is holding a packet of birth control pills between her teeth, with the comment, 'I love my contraceptives.' The image is an unconscious contradiction to her protest, voiced in *Meat Market*, against a culture that "tries to stamp itself all over one's womb and clamp itself around one's ovaries and shame XX-genotype women for owning bodies that can create new life."

The photo illustrates an article in which Penny writes, "The contraceptive pill is one of the most important inventions of the last three centuries, and doesn't damage the environment so much as the status quo."

A self-described Marxist Penny sees taking the pill as a rebellion against the status quo, by which we can assume she means a rebellion against male dominance and female oppression. She has swallowed the idea of pill taking as a liberating act.

She also fails to address the fact that the impact of synthetic hormones secreted into our waterways is significant to the reproductive health of many species, whether these come from industry, agriculture or the pill.

Penny describes the image in the article with the statement – "here I am nomming my tasty tasty oral contraceptives. Om nom nom."

Radical menstruation activists believe that the act of stopping and hiding our periods with hormonal contraceptives and sanitary products is a mark of corporate ownership over our bodies. To them, being open and honest about menstruation and critical of the prescription of hormonal contraceptives is an important element of establishing an identity that is independent of the pressures of consumerism. They encourage women to separate out what they want, feel and like from what they are pressured to choose and from there begin to construct their selves outside of the boundaries of what they are told is appropriate.

In a piece for xoJane entitled 'My Birth Control Gave Me A Mental Breakdown' Jessie Lochrie writes about the damage done to her mental health by the NuvaRing. The NuvaRing is increasingly popular with women in the US as it requires changing only once a month and is pushed as "low hormone." Lochrie describes, "One night at three or four AM, I shook my boyfriend awake, sobbing. I said, gasping for air, "I can't stop thinking about killing myself." The next day he announced that we were taking the Ring out. I protested wildly, saying that I was just adjusting, that the first few months were always a bit difficult. Until he mentioned it, it hadn't occurred to me at all that my sudden, severe change in mood was because of the birth control. We ended up in the bathroom, with him more or less pinning me down while he took the Ring out — I couldn't reach it myself, and I was so determined to keep it in, to really give it a try, that I would never have removed it on my own. I cried the entire time, of course."

The fact that even in the throws of a serious reaction to hormonal birth control women find it very difficult to relinquish them makes a strong argument for the addictive quality of these drugs.

In response to released research on the impact of naturally occurring estrogen and progesterone on traits of addiction, Dr Prior wrote an article titled 'Hooked On Estrogen.' The research concluded that estrogen assists with addictive behaviors. Dr Prior believes that menopausal hot flashes and night sweats are symptoms of estrogen addiction. Withdrawal from hormone therapy produces drug withdrawal-like problems. She sees one of the central issues with hormonal contraceptives as the creation of an estrogen-dominant state. "The animal evidence showing estrogen increases addictive behaviors is strong and extensive.

Hundreds of experiments show that female rats become addicted more quickly than male rats, are less likely to become addicted without their ovaries but the quick-dependence problem returns when they are given estrogen," she explains.

Dr Prior argues that Yaz and Yasmin (and all drospirenone-containing pills) have their particular impact because drospirenone is a weak progestin in comparison to those stronger progestins used in previous generations of pills and this allows the synthetic estrogen to dominate. The research shows that naturally occurring progesterone, and possibly bio-identical progesterone, can aid addiction recovery.

Many women find the decision to come off hormonal birth control much harder than a decision to change their diet or to take up a healthy habit. They are fearful of living without this addition to their bodies.

Our society is not ambivalent to this choice. A decision to try an alternative non-hormonal method of contraception is unsupported by the ideology. Women don't see the non-hormonal alternatives reflected by the culture. There are no signs that it is an option other women choose. There develops a physical and psychological dependency on the drugs that are bolstering our sense of what it means to be a woman in this world.

We are addicted to these drugs because we have come to believe that we need them. Our society assimilated hormonal contraception into its structure. To be compliant to the drugs is to be compliant to that structure.

Corsetry

"It is important not only that she wear rib-crushing garments but they she lace them up herself," Susan Faludi, *Backlash*.

A woman on the pill embodies the feminine ideal set out in the Victorian age. She is kept physically child-like. Women willingly slip into this established mold in the hope that they will be able to 'pass' – to reattribute a term used predominantly by the transgender community – in a society that idealizes the male. It is men that are the inspirational model.

Another interviewee from May's book remarks, "The Pill became a form of abuse. I would take it straight through for months at a time so as to miss my period and be able to have sex like a man."

The phrase "like a man" is nonsense of course, no more founded in reality than assumptions of how women behave. To have sex like a man translates as without emotion or attachment and with multiple partners. We believe men can have sex without fear of consequences. In a society that elevates sex as the source of self-knowledge and as a woman's path to liberation, to have sex with complete freedom is the ultimate goal. Yet it's doubtful that even men want to have sex "like a man" despite any desire for multiple partners or no fear of pregnancy.

Do men have sex without emotion and attachment any more than women? We are set against each other in order to remain isolated and better controlled.

Third wave feminism has established a "sex-positive" standpoint. In the US, being sex-positive is the logical position to take when faced with abstinence-only sex education and the puritanical hangover of a culture that can make itself crazy over Janet Jackson's breasts or obsess over Anthony Weiner's erection. Sex-positive feminism was borne out of the movement's detachment from those involved in policing pornography and those who believed women working in the sex industry to be solely victims of male coercion. Although striving for further inclusivity, sex-positive feminism alienates women who feel that the central message is that they should be having sex "like a man." Sex-positive feminism has the ability to sideline women as frigid, old-fashioned, and deluded followers of the socially acceptable. Can one be sexually liberated and in a monogamous heterosexual marriage? Not now it seems.

Levy writes in her New Yorker review of Wolf's *Vagina: A New Biography* that the sex-positive movement was established under the pressure of fear, "The woman as body trope had serious and worrisome implications: if a woman is necessarily irrational, hormonal, instinctual, and sensual, you don't want her running your company, let alone your country."

As we can see, hormonal is not a neutral term. Both men and women are hormonal in that they have hormones, which is all "hormonal" ought to logically mean. Levy continues, "The pro-sex feminists fell prey to the alluring but dubious conflation of fornication and emancipation. Orgasms are swell, but they are not the remedy to every injustice." Hormonal contraceptives were essential to the growth of this element of feminism.

The language used, such as women being "reduced" to their bodies, reveals that we believe women's bodies are naturally not as good as a men's bodies.

Life coach Miranda Gray's *The Optimized Woman: Using Your Menstrual Cycle to Achieve Success and Fulfillment* presents the idea that a woman's body is an untapped resource for the individual and society. She writes, "In a world where every business needs an edge to keep ahead, tapping into the vast resource of abilities women offer could provide the necessary inspired leaps to stay one step ahead of competitors." It is cycle tracking as self-help.

Gray asserts that women cannot practice self-improvement and reach their personal potential without acknowledging and honoring their cycle. Gray extrapolates this thought to suggest that society at large ought to take note of women's talents during different times of the month and actively capitalize on those, such as creativity and intuition, which tend to be ignored.

Although not a politically aware writer, Gray embarks on this education with the view that men and the male-dominant culture should and could welcome the female cycle's encroachment on the nine to five, five-day working week.

Instead of suppressing their biology to fit the system, women can use their biology to make capitalism work more effectively.

Her theories are dependent on a belief that being productive for the sake of the economy and becoming a successful capitalist is the ideal goal in life and the best way for women to spend their energies and time. The success and fulfillment of the title are only brought about via very narrow means.

Gray argues that women can use knowledge of their cycle to become more successful workers. She states, "We all know the saying that if we want to change the world we must first change ourselves. But what if we change during the month; does that mean the world changes too? Yes." Gray does not directly advocate for social or political change, but an evolution of the current system. Women may have felt that taking the pill allows them to be more successful in this male-dominated world, but Gray suggests women's own biology is the key to living a life of productivity.

Gray writes that if the emphasis were on productivity instead of attendance with flexible hours installed to allow women to work more hours at certain points in their cycle when their energy is high to make up for lost hours at other times then there would be no cause for concern. Gray is British and therefore has a somewhat different viewpoint on the working environment to the "at will" employee of the US system. Her book is grounded in essentialist teachings but repackaged for the modern Cosmopolitan-reading woman.

Gray's book includes a chapter for bosses on how to "get the best from women." Gray believes that if male bosses could understand the female cycle and approach women with their cycle in mind then they would garner more "positive" responses. Men can discover through a process of elimination or through providing four-fold options (to reflect the menstruation, ovulation and pre and post ovulation phases) as to how each task be approached. When there is no flexibility at work, Gray encourages women to benefit from their cycle in the choices they make in their home life and free time.

An interviewee describes how she has incorporated Gray's guide in to her management of her small business, "It makes work so much more enjoyable when you get to say, "That task doesn't resonate with where I am in my cycle, would you mind doing it instead."

This is reminiscent of the refrain captured most recently by the Occupy Movement from Melville's 'Bartleby, the Scrivener' – "I would prefer not to." A phrase said by a man who decides he no longer wants to do the dull work of copying legal documents.

On this Jonathan D. Greenberg, in an article for *The Atlantic*, writes, "To some sanguine temperaments," muses Melville's narrator, "it would be altogether intolerable.... I cannot credit that the mettlesome poet Byron would have contentedly sat down with Bartleby to examine a law document of, say five hundred pages, closely written in a crimpy hand." The invocation of Byron is crucial; Bartleby's writing is as far from poetry as you can get. It is bureaucratic scrivening, in which there is no room for originality, authorship, style, ornament, or pleasure. Is it any wonder that Bartleby "decide[s] upon doing no more writing"?"

Gray argues the same for women. During certain phases of the month women will also find dull repetitive work even more intolerable than during the rest of the month. At that time they should insist on doing a task more in tune with the talents being emphasized by their cycle. This is a strike, but tempered by the proposal that the boss will benefit in the long term by respecting the decision.

If we reason that women take hormonal contraceptives to fit into society and so not only for success, but for survival and self-preservation by belonging to and not standing separate from the majority, then we can see that Gray is offering an alternative avenue for women to fit without pharmaceuticals. By her teaching women are still bowing to patriarchal and capitalistic culture. She does not address those for whom being a better member of this system is not their aim, who want a positive relationship with their body for other reasons.

Self-improvement culture charges that if we change ourselves we can change our circumstances. It acknowledges there are problems but makes a bid to solve these problems through the individual. The individual must take responsibility for the problem and work actively to change it independently of others. In fact, self-help often encourages individuals not to expect the support or cooperation of others. It is about providing guides for people to navigate a society that is inhumane, discompassionate, and unconcerned with the physical and mental health of its members. The advice helps us make a place for ourselves in such a society. It helps us feel comfortable in a world that has only the comfort of the few in mind, and even they must not be satisfied with their lot.

Gray introduces a conflict between the masculine, socially sanctified "linear time" and feminine "cyclic" time.

Charles Eisenstein expands pertinently on Gray's implication that linear time is oppressive, "In effect, clocks turn time into another standardized, interchangeable part of the World Machine, facilitating the engineering of the world. Only time thus devalued is a conceivable object of commerce. Otherwise, who would sell their moments, each infinitely precious, for a wage? Who would reduce time, i.e. life, to mere money? Leibnitz' merciless phrase, "Time is money," encapsulates a profound reduction of the world and enslavement of the spirit. It is not surprising that the revolutionaries of Paris's 1830 July Revolution went around the city smashing its clocks. The fundamental purpose of clocks is not to measure time; it is to coordinate human activity. Aside from that it is a fiction, a pretense: as Thoreau said, "Time measures nothing but itself." Smashing the clocks represents a refusal to sell one's time, a refusal to schedule one's life or to bring it into conformity with the needs of specialized mass society."

Women are indoctrinated to strive for perfection. They are, as they understand it, inherently lacking and must compensate for this lack. Hormonal contraceptives have become a tool in this struggle for self-improvement. The control women can exert over their bodies is treated as a viable substitute for their lack of control over their position in society.

The pill prevents women from functioning at their optimal level of health. The vitamin and nutrient deficiency, the impact on the endocrine system, the flattening out of peaks in hormones, and the wearing away of every bodily system takes its toll over time. It is true that an "optimized woman" would be a woman not on hormonal birth control. An "optimized woman" would be one allowed to ovulate as her body dictates.

Gray describes the ovulation or "expressive phase" as "a wonderful phase, with feelings of joy and happiness, creativity and self-expression, confidence and fulfillment, altruism and love." According to Gray's proposal, women are being held back in the workplace, in education, and in relationships by not experiencing their cycles.

In terms of the woman as worker Gray says this time is the best for "supporting both projects and people through heart-to-heart meetings, team building, mediating compromises, negotiating win-win deals and networking." The expressive phase is "the Optimum Time to sell ourselves, our work and our product or service." She marks out ovulation as a time to connect with other people, collaborate and coordinate and the menstruation phase as a time for "deep connection to the Universe beyond everyday concerns" and the intuitive and imaginative.

Hormonal contraceptives have caused women to lose their jobs, their relationships, friendships and hindered them in achieving their goals. They've been held back from fulfilling their potential. They have been set on a path of questioning their own judgment and beliefs.

Third-wave feminism is concerned with liberating women sexually, allowing them to put their own pleasure first and feel no shame about their sexual preferences. Supporting women in becoming active agents of their own sexuality as opposed to objects of other's sexual desires is thought to be key in elevating women's status in society. Yet when it comes to a woman's hormonal cycle, we are ready to sacrifice that for what we are told are the tools needed for spontaneous, unhindered sex – hormonal contraceptives.

Knowing your body, charting your cycle, is not just for women in committed relationships. To know when you're fertile should be seen as essential for those women desiring no-strings-attached sex. A woman can use a condom for protection from STIs but know with confidence from her own personal reading of her body that she can not get pregnant at that time.

Combined with an unsuppressed sex drive and emotional well-being - what could be more liberating?

As Katie Singer, author of *The Garden of Fertility* has noted, "I'm dreaming now: of adolescents knowing how their reproductive systems work before becoming sexually active and before they choose a birth control method; of men and women being as aware of our fertility as we are our sexuality."

Beyond female

In order for us to be able to honestly and openly discuss that the pill negatively impacts women it must be acknowledged that female biology is important. Such a discussion cannot avoid the claim that female bodies are different from male bodies. By arguing that a drug changes female biology and negatively impacts mood specifically, it must be admitted that our experience of life is connected to our biology. It is necessarily claimed that who we are is linked to our biology. To say that the ovulatory cycle, a specifically female bodily system, can not be shut down and ignored without serious repercussion, because it is vitally important to women's health is to run the risk of inciting the furor of those who feel they have fought long and hard to wrestle down and defeat the connection between women and their bodies. Such statements are controversial. Even using the word 'female' can be contentious today.

Bobel discusses in her work the idea of "smashing the binary." To her, this means doing away with the concepts of man and woman. The radical menstruation activists she interviews use the term "menstruators" in place of "women." In response Bobel asks how useful is the act of breaking down these gender boundaries when there is still so much discrimination faced by women just for being "women"?

She wonders whether it helps to say male and female are social constructs and go from there or whether, seeing as we do not yet live in a post-gender world, by doing this we are making too much of a leap and leaving a necessary struggle, and many women, behind.

In regards to the pill, we need to talk about "women" and "femaleness" because this is integral to how and why the pill came to exist and why it is still taken by so many women.

To say that the pill can change the way a woman feels by meddling with her biology reads as anti-feminist. It is also anti-feminist to not take women at their word and validate their personal experience by acknowledging it to be right and true.

Taking the pill might be seen as an act of trying to get beyond femaleness. As femaleness in our culture is understood in the negative, escaping its confines is good and progressive. Any dislike we develop of being female and of having a female body is rooted in the history of female bodies being seen as problematic and in need of male control.

In a televised advert for the brand a group of women, shown singularly one after the other, asks 'Who says you have to have twelve periods a year?' This defiant statement 'Who says?' is repeated a number of times. The authority that is being questioned here is unclear; as Kissling highlights it could be other women, men, the pharmaceutical industry, feminists, or even "your mother." The advert however suggests these women are rebelling against an authority by choosing Seasonique. These women are overcoming their biology and as such their femaleness.

This drug is not just birth control; it is, as a Yaz tagline once explained "beyond birth control."

Taking these drugs is about being 'beyond female.' Female, as this advert suggests, is not good, female is not something you want, female needs to be controlled, influenced, changed and organized into something neater, easier and less frightening to you and those around you.

When we take the pill we shut down the interior indicators of our femaleness. The exterior remains and it is this that makes it acceptable. In actuality, the pill makes women more physically attractive within the boundaries of our Western patriarchal capitalist culture. We are free of messy periods, we may have clearer skin, be slimmer, we may have bigger breasts, and we are supposedly rid of troublesome PMS.

The former YazXpress area of Bayer's promotional Yaz website asked women to 'Get with the program!' Women taking or interested in taking Yaz were able to sign up for an "insider's guide to Yaz, fashion, music and style." The articles in this guide were co-created by the magazine editors at Elle and Cosmopolitan, the pages of which frequently feature print adverts for birth control brands. Yaz was associated with an affluent, glamorous way of life. Taking Yaz would lead to the life of an attractive, confident 'Sex And The City' type of woman. Coolness, sexiness, modernity and glamour were linked to taking this brand.

In 2009 Bayer took on Lo Bosworth, star of *The Hills*, a popular Los Angeles-based reality show about a group of twenty-something women aspiring to make it in Hollywood, as a spokeswoman for Yaz in Canada. Of her support for the drug, Bosworth remarked, "As a 'Gen Yer' working in the entertainment industry, I need to be disciplined. I need to make sure I'm taking care of myself so nothing interrupts my day."

The pill has long been linked with the women's liberation movement. The aforementioned Seasonique advert splits an act of rebellion from any concept of the collective and makes liberation something purely individualistic and inward looking.

Although certain procedures have entered the mainstream in the US, women who have plastic surgery can come up against much criticism. Discussion circles around ideas of women taking plastic surgery choices too far, getting obsessed with making changes, making choices based on their insecurities or in response to difficult experiences such as the failing career and the bad break up. A woman who chooses to undergo plastic surgery is choosing to change her body. She is exerting control over her body. She is choosing to be 'beyond' human through changing her very physicality. She is choosing to not age or not submit to what her genes, her biology, have given her.

How does plastic surgery factor under the women's liberation message of "my body, my choice" and why is so much said about the psychological and social impacts of this choice?

Why are people who have lots of plastic surgery a concern, but not people who take a drug to shut down their ovulatory cycle, stop their periods and 'perfect' their bodies from the inside out?

When using Yasmin people often commented on my perfected, flawless skin and its "doll-like" appearance.

We are used to seeing labels for "BPA-free" plastics as we have become more aware of the synthetic estrogens in many everyday plastic products. One study shows seventy percent of items made of plastic leach chemicals that act like estrogen.

The perfected body, as our ideology teaches, is not female but male. If we shut down the essential biological center of femaleness, the primary sexual characteristics, then can we say that women on the pill are still "female"? The mythology of the pill reveals how femininity is valued within our society. Women on the pill still have their secondary sexual characteristics. We understand judgment and valuation of our femininity is directly correlated with our appearance, significantly our attractiveness. Women who are not attractive by the Western cultural standards have their femaleness questioned, as do women who have less defined visual secondary sexual characteristics, such as smaller breasts or a wider waistline or shorter legs. The ideal body in this age of plastic surgery has exaggerated exterior signs of femininity.

In a piece for the *Vice* magazine website, porn actress Stoya writes on her experience choosing a birth control method. She admits she feels hormonal contraceptives are the best choice for an actress having sex with men but states, "the pill and I don't seem to get along well." After suffering with side effects in her teens Stoya had not considered using the pill again until she began performing in scenes with men. She started taking the latest brand, "Four months into taking Yaz, I was miserable. I bled profusely the whole time. Instead of migraines once or twice a month, I had them multiple times a week. I had intense mood swings and was constantly dizzy. I had planned on giving it another one or two months, hoping that my body would adjust, and then I fainted while waiting in line at the bank."

She came off Yaz and four years later decided to try Ortho Tricyclen Lo, but only lasted three months. She now takes Loestrin 24 Fe and still experiences continuous bleeding and mood swings but describes how pleased she is with one particular side effect – an increase in the size of her breasts, "Dragging myself out of bed became a herculean effort, and the idea of showering or brushing my teeth was beyond my abilities. Everything felt tragic and hopeless. My only redeeming qualities were my tits.

They were by no means giant hooters, but they were noticeably fuller, which was pretty cool. I started to think hormonal birth control was a patriarchal plot to keep women down by rendering us completely loony. The question, "How can we ever break the glass ceiling, if we can't stop crying?" actually came out of my mouth. I still feel nuts, but hey… at least this B-cup kind of fits." Stoya has self-awareness and insight into her situation but she sacrifices her health and well-being partly, it seems, because she's not aware of the alternatives or feels they are off-limits to her. She wryly jokes about her predicament.

A woman on the pill is likely to experience low libido and will certainly feel some detachment from her sexuality. The feeling of sexuality is different from female sexuality, but is vitally important, as it is personal to women and separate from their relationships to men. Not feeling sexual could lead to a desire to look exaggeratedly sexual and to appear and behave very sexually in an act of over-compensation. Such a desire can be fulfilled in part through plastic surgery.

Transgender teen boys take hormonal contraceptives in a bid to slow the appearance of their male maturation in pubic hair, vocal changes and the development of the masculine body shape. The pill is self-prescribed as a treatment for their situation and is more readily available and cheaper than the hormone treatments that can be bought online or prescribed by a doctor. The pill can be taken from sisters, mothers and friends.

Transgender women, and men, take hormone treatments in order to fit into society by physically adhering to the require-ments of acceptable female and male bodies. Some transgender activists speculate as to whether they would choose to undergo hormone treatments, and particularly surgery, if it weren't for the requirements set out by the culture. They consider whether they make these choices for themselves (some feel they do, for their own mental and physical health) or for those around them.

Penny asserts in *Meat Market* that trans women understand

that "socially acceptable female identity is something that must be purchased and imposed artificially on the flesh."

We support modifying and suppressing our bodily functions with science to perfect our faulty bodies even when we are generally healthy and well, and even when the notion of what it means to be faulty is so spurious. When experiencing the side effects from hormonal contraceptives women have a tendency to blame what they view as their own overly hormonal, unpredictable, difficult bodies that in reacting negatively to these drugs are behaving badly. It is their bodies that are not good enough for the drugs.

Even if we are not ill, science is making us better. We are becoming better humans, better women.

Statins might make us less "faulty" or less likely to have high cholesterol, but in what other ways do and will these drugs make us ill? In what other ways can we deal with this human faultiness that is not long-term drug use that impacts the whole body?

The pill is no longer about birth control; it is about being a better, improved woman.

The terms 'healthiness' or 'healthy' might be viewed as oppressive. They suggest healthy bodies that are experiencing natural ovulation cycles are the norm, and as such superior than perceived 'unhealthy' bodies - those bodies not experiencing cycles. The physical norm promoted in our culture is a period-free, PMS-free body. Periods are an abnormal event. They are so abnormal women are convinced it is not natural for them to even have periods.

If there is in fact no physical norm in that all women's bodies are different and healthiness cannot be associated with such a concept, then there is no reference point for sickness and we can all claim disability. Menstruation and the hormone cycle have long been presented as disabling for women both mentally and physically. This reasoning has been used as justification for the oppression of women.

Pharmaceutical companies move the target constantly from birth control to menstruation suppression, from acne control to mood control and in so doing they are betraying their motivations. By medicalizing the normal physiology of the female body, and saying overtly that it needs to be controlled and improved upon they are betraying the foundations of pill promotion.

If we believe we should get beyond our femaleness we are accepting that women's bodies are bad and need to be made good. The consumer economy is crafty; it will always find an avenue for assimilation. The pharmaceutical companies are listening at the door to our presumed post-feminist talk.

Section Five: The Drug Pushers

"Pills are to sell, not to take. If we put horse manure in a capsule we could sell it to 95% of these doctors." Harry Lloynd, former president of Parke-Davis, a subsidiary company of Pfizer (*The Doctor's Case Against The Pill*, Barbara Seaman)

"I developed fairly bad acne at age seventeen and the doctor told me to try Diane. A few months after taking it I became irrationally irritable, I would snap at my family, cry uncontrollably, and had immense fatigue. I began having problems focusing at school. I had always been a happy, optimistic, and sociable person, but on the pill I became anxious and depressed. After three years I decided to get off the pill and my mind cleared, my mood lifted, I felt so much lighter and more able to handle things. Last summer when I decided to try Alesse as I was starting a new relationship. I immediately felt a difference. I went back to feeling tired all day long, regardless of how much sleep I got, I was unreasonable and quick-tempered, but also guilt-ridden and anxious. As a result of all the anxiety, I developed moderate adrenal fatigue. I was a completely healthy teenager with just some pimples and I was given a pill that robbed me of my emotional stability and mental health for years. Every time I went to the doctor, they attributed my difficulties to my life. I am enraged that my doctor jumped directly to giving me contraception for a skin issue and that other contraceptive options are rarely presented to women as viable alternatives to the pill." – Danielle

The push and the pull

For Damien Hirst's installation entitled 'Pharmacy' the walls are fitted with glass-fronted cases filled with medications of all kinds. A desk is lined with apothecary bottles in bright colors. Three plates of honey and honeycomb sit on stools that form a triangle in the room's center.

The honey lures the insects that in all of Hirst's work are representatives for people and these insects are then churned through and killed by the Insect-O-Cutor. Of 'Pharmacy,' Hirst has said, "I can't understand why most people believe in medicine and don't believe in art, without questioning either." 'Pharmacy' casts doubt over our faith in pharmaceuticals to stave off death and promote life. The work draws parallels between the uncritical trust put in religious doctrine and the trust in the medical industry.

We are drawn to medications not only for survival but for all that they promise through progress, immortality and the improvement of the human body.

Those drugs that people that are otherwise healthy take are even more of a matter of faith for their users than those drugs taken to prevent immediate pain or illness. We will all die, Hirst is saying, regardless of the reduction of the risks of living. Sometimes the drugs we take with the belief of improving and extending our existence are killing us faster or ruining our experience of life.

Hirst's work also brings to mind the use of thought manipulation in science. Studies that have shown the significant impact of placebos that are provided to patients with a positive recommendation from their doctors. Direct-to-consumer advertising and consultations with doctors create a sermonizing effect around pharmaceuticals. Women will believe Yaz, the Nuvaring or Mirena are good for them if they are taking in messages that encourage them to think of it as a miracle cure. The impact of positive affirmation is strong. If a drug is promoted as perfect its users find it hard to be critical of that drug even if their own experience would suggest the opposite.

The birth control pill is a $22 billion a year industry with approximately sixty brands on the market. Hormonal contraceptives are often a long-term commitment; a woman may take one brand or different brands for up to four decades. If she takes the pill this can cost as much as $80 a month in the US for someone without health insurance.

Pharmaceutical companies collectively spent $5 billion on direct to consumer advertising in 2006, an eighty percent increase from 2002. It is more profitable to create new drugs that are only slightly different from the drugs that are already available and market these well than to create "new" drugs. For every dollar spent on basic research, $19 goes to advertising and marketing. One study suggested that overall pharmaceutical companies spent twice as much on marketing as research.

Eighty percent of people who see drug adverts remembered a drug's benefits, while only twenty percent can recall the side effects. Rapid speech rates and using visual and auditory distractions during the reeling off of potential side effects makes it harder for us to process this information.

The market for lifestyle drugs is currently worth $23 billion – lifestyle drugs include statins, hypertensives and decongestants.

In an article for *Alternet* Martha Rosenberg writes on the '15 Dangerous Drugs Big Pharma Shoves Down Our Throats.' Drugs such as Lipitor, Ambien and Yaz are examples of "the FDA approving once-unapprovable drugs by transferring risk onto the public's shoulders with "we warned you" labels," she writes, "The warnings are supposed to make people make their own safety decisions. Except that people just think FDA wouldn't have approved it if it weren't safe." Lipitor is the best-selling drug in the world because it can be prescribed to those at real risk of heart attack plus those who only fear the possibility of developing a risk of heart attack. Rosenberg quotes a Tennessee ophthalmologist, "My older patients literally do without food so that they can buy these medicines that make them sicker, feel bad, and do nothing to improve life."

We are, as Rosenberg suggests, merely acting as test subjects who are paying for the privilege instead of being paid.

The American College of Obstetricians' 2012 guidelines state that the implant and the IUD should be the first choices for doctors providing contraception to teens. The organization emphasized the safety and effectiveness of these methods. It recommends in the report that doctors discuss these methods with teens at the forefront of their conversations about pregnancy prevention. This report set up long-acting contraceptive methods as the decided future of birth control for women. Liberal and progressive parents are given the go-ahead to be put their teen on a LARC and as such send them what they believe to be a sex-positive message.

Insurance companies can make their own decision as to which and how many contraceptive options are available to their members. In similarity to the NHS the push for efficiency and the lack of one-to-one care makes hormonal contraceptives an easy option. Branded drugs will sometimes be charged with a co-pay, which will perhaps send more women towards the generic brand with the same synthetic hormones. The patents on some hormonal contraceptives like the patch, IUD and the ring won't expire for some time and therefore there are no currently available generic versions. Varieties of delivery methods are pharmaceutical companies attempt at rehashing the same technology to create a new opportunity for patenting and bigger profits.

Women, however, often do feel uncomfortable switching to a generic drug and some have taken to online forums to complain of side effects experienced as a result of such a swap. Although the drugs are comprised of the same synthetic hormones women may blame side effects they are experiencing from build up of the use of the drug on the swap instead of the drugs themselves. Of course, there is an element here of that faith in pharmaceuticals. Brands engender more faith than generics because they are surrounded by positive affirmations through advertising. Generic brands do not carry those messages despite having the same medical impact.

What might be seen is an increased uptake of IUD use to match this method's popularity in Europe. The copper ParaGard IUD does not inhibit ovulation, whereas the hormonal Mirena IUD does, although to what extent is in constant debate. Currently just 8.5% of women in the US use these methods, partly due to the checkered past of the Dalkon Shield device and partly due to an unease with the procedure for insertion. In France and Norway, for example, twenty-five percent of women on birth control use IUDs, but most European countries have seen the hormonal Mirena outstrip the ParaGard. In China, a full forty-one percent use a version of the copper IUD, partly due to the one-child policy of the government and partly as a result of coercion by that government.

Eldridge describes how women in the US are pressured to take the Mirena over the ParaGard. There is financial pressure from the pharmaceutical company Bayer placed on doctors and clinics. The Mirena costs several hundred dollars more than the ParaGard and lasts just five years instead of ten. Unlike the ParaGard, the Mirena produces light; shorter periods for some women and can even stop periods entirely. The ParaGard marketing makes use of its difference, staking claim in the fact that it is "hormone free" and "won't interfere with your natural menstrual cycle." Yet the methods are often lumped together in media reportage and discussions, with an effect of downplaying the role of the hormones in the Mirena and suggesting the only impact of these hormones is to lighten or completely eliminate bleeding.

Yet the internet is awash with women claiming the Mirena has caused them some serious emotional and physical problems. The symptoms of withdrawal after the device is removed are so well-known amongst its users they have named this time and its impact "The Mirena Crash."

Towards the end of 2012 lawsuits began to mount against Bayer in regards to Mirena. The claims of negligence assert that Bayer is intentionally selling a dangerous product by the means of deceptive, aggressive marketing. The law suits focus on the life-threatening risks of ectopic pregnancy, uterus perforation, migration of the device and pelvic inflammatory disease. In a prominent TV advertising campaign Bayer claimed the Mirena would make women "look and feel great" and have improved intimacy and sex with their partner.

In 2013 Bayer will release the Skyla IUD in the US, with plans to release the device in Europe under the name Jaydess. The device emits the same synthetic hormone as the Mirena, but is smaller in size. Skyla lasts three years to the Mirena's five-year expiration date. It is aimed at teen and young women. Although it has been said that the Mirena is suitable for women who have not had children, it was previously promoted as only available for women who had children. The launch of Skyla is an obvious move to sidestep this potential market-narrowing confusion.

RH Reality Check responded to this news with an article hyperbolically titled, 'Could New Intrauterine Contraception Skyla Help Women Reach For The Stars,' walking a thin line between journalism and PR.

The ParaGard copper-based IUD works in two ways. One, the IUD is a foreign object and the body reacts to it immunologically as for any foreign object, by attacking it. This attack creates an inflammatory response. Chronic inflammation is detrimental to health in general and in particular suppresses immune function. Two, the copper changes the metabolic balance associated with fertility.

The ParaGard may be hormone-free but it is still reliant on medical intervention and doctors often do not understand the full extent of its potential impacts. There are reports, for example, of the ParaGard producing copper toxicity. The imbalances that can occur as a result of the increase in copper and the whole body response to inflammation can open a woman up to increased infections. The thyroid and adrenal glands and nervous system are very sensitive to copper imbalances and this can cause a myriad of emotional and neurological problems. Changed levels of copper can cause zinc deficiency and zinc is essential to many bodily systems.

Many women turn to the copper IUD after becoming disillusioned with hormonal birth control without realizing it can potentially cause some similar health problems.

As well as holding their own set of potential side effects, there are issues that set LARCs apart from the pill. It might be some time before women will take up these methods over the pill but their implementation for the young suggests the persuasive push will make them the first talking point in the doctor's office.

If a woman has paid highly for such a device she is yet more likely to doubt her decision to not continue with it, as she will possibly feel pressured to make the most of her investment. If the insurance company has paid for her, then she will have a hard time finding support for its removal.

On this Wershler writes, "The Affordable Care Act requires all health plans issued on or after August 1, 2012 to provide no-charge access to FDA-approved LARCs. What's it going to take to convince health-care providers to remove an expensive contraceptive, provided for "free," that was supposed to last for three to 10 years?"

These "forget-about-it" forms of contraception provide an opportunity for women to detach their experience entirely from the device. If health issues appear one year or five years into use, as they sometimes do due on the build up effect and the woman's changing and aging body, then she is less likely to consider they are caused by a device designed precisely for her to be unconscious of its presence. Women already have difficulty associating the pill with their health problems, but these devices actively promote that disconnect. Of course, promoting them as "forget-about-it" options also downplays the possibility of experiencing negative effects. Yet for some women the change to their body is so obvious it is hard to ignore.

LARCs make hormonal birth control use a norm and seal their role in every young woman's life. Long-term devices will be present in a woman's body even when she is not sexually active. LARCs confirm hormonal contraception as a treatment for being a young woman regardless of your actual need for pregnancy prevention.

The application of continuous hormones without any breaks over years means women are taking in more synthetic hormones over each year – twenty-five percent more. New progestins used in the NuvaRing, Implanon, Mirena and third generation birth control pills like Yaz are under-researched. Women are taught to equate less hormones (such as pills with "low" or "lo" in the name or those presented as having a low hormone dose) as better for their body in a style that has similarities to a dedicated smoker's perception of low-tar or light cigarettes.

Research is emerging that argues starting teens on hormonal contraceptives has serious knock-on health effects in later years including a staggering fifty percent increased risk of developing breast cancer.

In the US doctors can be as influenced by direct-to-consumer televised and print advertising of drugs as their patients. They also have to contend with drug company representatives who visit their surgery peddling their company's latest drug and trying to get doctors to hawk the most expensive brands. These representatives use bribery – a vacation, dinner or cash bonuses – to get the doctors to work with them. It is common for drug companies to provide kickbacks and rewards to doctors if they push their pills, especially for off-label uses that widen the potential market. Pharmaceutical companies have spent billions of dollars in settlement payments to avoid admitting this relationship to the public. They benefit highly from our trust in doctors.

Doctors will say that having a relationship with the drug makers helps them understand the drugs better and allows them to provide more information to their patients. They can deny the influence of the money on their decision-making. They act as consultant, spokesperson or panel member at conferences sponsored by a drug company and provide the assurance of a medical practitioner in a corporate setting to help the delivery of a new pharmaceutical.

The New York Times conducted research that showed a quarter of doctors take cash payments from companies and that two-thirds accept gifts of lunches and dinners. *The Times* asserted this caused doctors to practice medicine differently – particularly encouraging them to prescribe drugs in "risky and unapproved" ways.

Tens of thousands of physicians are paid to promote drugs and provide information to drug companies to aid them in improving their marketing techniques. They are in a position to find out what women want, and why and then target their drugs to these needs regardless of the health consequences. This is not only an issue in the US, but also prevalent practice in the UK and Europe. Bringing doctors that accept such bribes to trial to examine the influence of this behavior is difficult as a jury fielded from the general public might be wary of criticizing a medical practitioner. Doctors are still imbibed with a large amount of faith by their patients and not treated like the service providers of any other industry.

President Obama mandated a new law in 2012 that will require pharmaceutical companies to name which doctors have received payments from them for consulting, travel, entertainment, research or speaking at events. The motivation is not only to provide a transparency to the patient but also to bring down costs as currently doctors are pushed to provide the most expensive, branded treatments.

Leonore Tiefer is Clinical Associate Professor of Psychiatry at the New York University School of Medicine and Albert Einstein College of Medicine. She has written widely about the medicalization of female sexuality and heads up the New View Campaign, which is a grassroots network challenging the distorted and oversimplified understanding of sexuality promoted by the pharmaceutical industry as a means to profit.

She is particularly involved in criticism of the race to produce a 'female Viagra.' The female Viagra patch Intrinsa was rejected by the FDA in 2004, not due on potential side effects but due on questions as to its results. Tiefer remarks on this, "For Intrinsa, and for Viagra, the placebo has shown to be extremely effective in clinical trials. The placebo provides a forty percent improvement. The drug itself showed an improvement higher than this, but not significantly. The pharmaceutical companies do not make direct comparison, because, as they say, they're not marketing the placebo."

The drug Flibanserin was in research until 2010. The aim was to treat women who lack libido and sexual desire. It was set up in opposition to hormonal birth control methods with their negative impact on libido. Dr Irwin Goldstein is very vocal about the negative effect of hormonal contraceptives on sexual desire. He has discussed openly the emotional and mental side effects of hormonal birth control. He's conducted studies to show that women are less interested in sex when on the pill. Yet he labels these issues as a dysfunction called "hypoactive sexual desire disorder" and is a strong supporter and bank rolled associate of the pharmaceutical company behind Flibanserin.

Goldstein has gone as far as to state that this drug would provoke "the beginning of an era for women," and that releasing it on the market would be a "unique and historic opportunity for women in the US and for the FDA." Research was halted when studies discovered it had very little impact beyond that of the comparative placebo pills. It also produced, of course, a myriad of side effects.

The documentary *Orgasm Inc* explores the pharmaceutical industry's involvement in developing disorders that can be responded to with the creation of a pill. The potential markers of disorders are widened to provide a broad spectrum of potential customers for a new drug. Just as hormonal contraceptives are now readily prescribed for an extensive list of health problems, a pill for sexual dysfunction will demand the creation of problems where there are only healthy variations on normal biological functions.

Orgasm Inc followed a middle-aged woman who became involved in the research testing of a female Viagra-type drug because she didn't realize that not being able to orgasm through penetration alone was not "abnormal." She assumed the drug was created to address this "problem."

As the New View Campaign outlines in its manifesto – it has become a requirement that a woman have sexual responses "like a man." The efforts to produce drugs are rooted in a standard that sets male sexuality as the norm, as a state to which women must aspire. The convenient, non-obstructive hormonal methods of birth control are means to allowing women to have sex "like a man."

The impact of hormonal contraceptives on many women has been exploited by the pharmaceutical industry. Instead of this issue causing us to question why we are happy for women to take a pill to have supposedly worry-free sex that denigrates their enjoyment of the act, we have a new range of medically-defined disorders for the DSM that instigate a new pill to solve the problems.

In 2009 Bayer announced it would be working on drugs to treat "symptoms" of menopause and other "gynecological disorders." Such disorders are defined as pelvic pain, vulvo-dynia and vaginitis. Vulvodynia is often experienced as pain during sex. Vaginitis is irritation or pain within the vagina.

A decrease in libido is just one of the pill's direct impacts on women's sexual desire and enjoyment. Hormonal birth control can thin the vaginal walls and cause tearing. There can be a decrease in natural lubrication and a decrease in the ability to orgasm. Dr. Andrew Goldstein, director of the US-based Centers for Vulvovaginal Disorders and one of the foremost vulvodynia experts in North America blames an increase in complaints of this kind on lower dose, new generation pills. Dr Goldstein has suggested women consider the cause of these issues is their hormonal contraceptive or any other hormone-based treatment they've been receiving before they take another action to alleviate the symptoms.

Often pain during sex and other "gynecological disorders" are diagnosed as the result of psychological issues with sexual contact, as the symptom of an STI or the product of "rough" sexual encounters. Those women who experience these problems and are not on hormonal contraceptives are often prescribed the birth control pill as the treatment in another example of its status as a "cure-all" drug.

Slate highlighted the work of microbiologist Gregor Reid in an article that outlined how his research makes the case for vaginosis presenting a threat to reproduction. Vaginitis is one kind of vaginosis, which is essentially the growth of bacteria and development of a pH imbalance in the vagina. The ensuing inflammation can, Reid believes, prevent fertilization of an egg, cause spontaneous abortion and provoke pre-term births. As said, the pill produces vaginitis and suppresses the immune system. According to the article thirty percent of women in the US have a type of vaginosis.

Eldridge argues that instead of moving forward with slightly modified versions of hormonal contraceptives and differing delivery methods we should be reconsidering whether what seemed right for women over fifty years ago may not be right for women today.

Using her research into hormonal therapy for menopause for comparison, Eldridge writes, "Hormone therapy and estrogen therapy were on the market for sixty years before conventional wisdom about those medications was overturned. There is still much we don't know about the pill and because of limitations on the type of research we can do, much we may never know."

In 2009 Bayer stated too that they are looking to open up the Asia-Pacific markets for sales of their birth control pills as well as their other hormonal contraceptive devices like the Mirena. Hormonal contraceptives are not popular amongst women in China, India, Vietnam or Japan.

Currently In the United States, 80 percent of women born after 1945 have used the pill. In Western Europe 50 percent of married women use the pill. Yet, in Japan the pill was not legalized until the end of the 1990s. There eighty percent of women use condoms as their form of contraception. It has been assumed that Japanese women's disinterest in hormonal contraceptives is due on the country's presumed restrictions on women's social freedoms. However, there are reports that Japanese women show more concern over the side effects and dislike taking on the full burden of pregnancy prevention.

Only 1.3% of Japanese women using contraception take the pill. Three years after it was legalized seventy percent of women reported they would never consider using it.

Although abortions are not as contentious an issue in Japan as in the US, the US has a higher rate of abortion whereas Japan shows a similar rate to that of the UK. There are reports that suggest fertility awareness methods, although not necessarily those that incorporate all three signs of fertility, are popular in Japan with more women being aware of their ovulatory time and using this knowledge to avoid pregnancy. The calendar rhythm method, its invention in part attributed to a Japanese doctor, is popular. It uses mathematical calculation based on the pattern of a woman's previous cycles to predict days of fertility. It is far less effective than fertility awareness methods that determine the days of fertility based on real time observations of the signs of fertility.

Condoms are marketed creatively in Japan, they are readily available and, perhaps most importantly, the technology has been improved to create condoms with a better feel and performance. Condom brands Crown and Beyond Seven utilize Sheerlon instead of latex and have a different fit and feel to popular US brands. They are considered the height of condom technology in strength, sensitivity and stretch.

Anthropology professor at the University of Virginia Allison Alexy has written on the subject of Japanese women's relationship to hormonal contraceptives. "The portrayal of Japanese culture in the Western media is simplified and ignorant," she states. "The Japanese are often represented as robotic collectivists who have no sense of individualism. Japanese women in particular are said to be living in the 1970s still in terms of social standing. This just isn't true."

Alexy explains that Japanese women have concerns about what the birth control pill could potentially do to their bodies. They feel that the drug makers have not researched the impact fully. They also don't believe that women should be burdened with the sole responsibility of contraception.

The common mainstream analysis of their disinterest in hormonal contraceptives argues that Japanese women are socially oppressed and not encouraged by their doctors or government to use these methods because the government desires to keep liberation from them. But Alexy asks, "What is our definition of liberation for women from this assumption?" She argues that, "Japanese women's concerns about side effects are very much valid. To not be pressured to take hormonal contraceptives by your partner and your society, that is liberating. A man can use a condom and it has no impact on his body.

Isn't it a sign of their liberation that their partners offer to use condoms and that they can have that mutual agreement in regards to contraception?"

This agreement is based partly on the different cultural view of intimacy. In the US condoms are seen as the protection that you use with strangers or while dating around and once in a steady relationship you move on to unprotected sex. Sex without a condom in this context is romanticized. Using a condom with your long term boyfriend or husband is believed to suggest a lack of trust in their fidelity. In Japan the opposite view holds, women see a man using condoms as a demonstration of his affection. The condom might diminish his pleasure somewhat but he'd rather make that sacrifice than ask his partner to take a drug.

In Japan if a man loves you enough he will offer to use a condom.

The context in which this situation can develop is specific to Japan. Although a world economic power, Japan has a very low birth rate and a rapidly aging population. Women and men marry late (thirty-one and thirty-two respectively) and only three percent of children are born outside of wedlock, compared to approximately forty-five percent in the US. The majority of abortions in Japan are conducted before eleven weeks due to accessibility and the relative affordability of the procedure. A significant number of the women seeking an abortion are married and already have children. Although abortions are socially acceptable Japan still holds a low to medium rate of procedures when viewed in comparison to the rest of the world.

Tiana Norgren argues in *Abortion Before Birth Control* that although limiting the number of children a family is, in the US and Europe, important for the consumer economy, in Japan a higher birth rate is needed to sustain growth. Not backing hormonal contraceptives is, she believes, a tactical move by the Japanese government. Norgren also puts forth the idea that abortion services provide certain sectors of society with much money and those sectors have enough power to push back against hormonal contraceptives. Although, she admits, the primary obstacle has clearly been women's suspicion of the potential side effects.

Norgren's approach to investigating this situation is illuminating. Coming from a perspective that advocates and champions the pill as the most logical, modern and civilized method of birth control she reveals very clearly some of the nonsensical reasoning that underlines the West's acceptance of hormonal contraceptives as the one and only way. Through struggling with the Japanese cultural concern over the health impact of the pill and contrasting the perspective to other countries that are suggested to be more enlightened, she brings into focus the close to negligent attitude that prevails in the US when it comes to women's health.

In Norgren's opinion it is paternalistic to prevent women from using the pill by making it illegal for contraceptive purposes. Her suggestion is that the pill's availability in the US is evidence of a lack of paternalism by the government and medical establishment. Norgren is critical of Japanese officials putting national interests, specifically the problem of falling birth rates, before individual women's needs without acknowledging that happily pill-popping countries do just the same.

Norgren repeatedly states the safety of second and third generation birth control pills as better than that of legal abortion when, in the US, death occurs in 0.0006% of all legal surgical abortions (one in 160,000 cases). She argues that once the pill was approved in Japan the medical establishment insisted that women using the drug have check-ups every three months including a pelvic exam as a form of subtle "propaganda" to suggest to women that the pill is a potentially dangerous drug. What little morality-based debate there has been over abortion she claims to be a pharmaceutical industry-led conspiracy to boost pill sales.

In Japan the limitation of abortion access is only good news for the makers of medical contraceptives who see this as widening their market. Norgren does not ask if this might in fact be the same case in the US.

With seventy-two percent of women saying they have concerns about side effects for the pill, Norgren remarks that it has been said that it is easier for a woman to admit to having an abortion than to say she is on the pill.

Why are women so reluctant to take the pill when Japan is the second largest pharmaceutical market in the world with the second highest consumption of pharmaceuticals per capita?

Norgren is baffled by an interviewee who suggests: "Japanese women prefer methods that interfere less with the natural rhythms of the woman's body," and in response to turns to the thesis of *Is Menstruation Obsolete?* The concern and interest of Japanese midwives is reduced to an economic issue. Norgren argues that they only protested the legalization of the pill because they cannot sell it to their patients like they can condoms and diaphragms. The message of her work is clear - Japanese women are fools for not taking up the pill with enthusiasm like the rest of the world's civilized societies.

An entire book could be dedicated to this US-Japan comparison alone. Obviously the availability of social support services impact on the abortion rate of a country. *The New York Times* ran a report on the problems faced specifically by Japanese women trying to balance children and careers. The work requirements of the Japanese culture in which very long hours are demanded of employees mean couples cannot add to their family without serious consideration. Overwork is such a problem in Japan that a death due to the extreme exertion has its own name – "karoshi."

Being patient

Five months into writing my blog I received an email from a drug compliance officer from Bayer. She asked if we could speak on the phone. When we did, she wanted to know where I had seen reports of the side effects of Yasmin. I directed her to the websites, including the Yaz Survivors forum. She remarked that even though, as I pointed out, they were "the most complained about drugs on the internet," these testimonies weren't enough to necessitate any kind of action on the company's part and could easily be dismissed as coincidental. She suggested that instead of writing about my problems with these drugs in a public space that I disclose them privately to the FDA who would certainly take action if it were considered necessary.

The idea of "non-compliance" to a drug suggests a certain brand loyalty. "The pill" is a brand in the way the Hoover is a brand or Xerox or Kleenex.

An intriguing reaction of the medical industry to non-compliance is an increase in research into potential predictors of women's negative response to pills. The acknowledgment that each woman's body is different, each hormone cycle is different and that despite the varieties of dosages available, some women will report side effects on every pill is a step forward. Each woman does not require the same dose of synthetic hormones to prevent ovulation. Research is underway into individualizing prescriptions of synthetic hormones.

These realms of research do not appear to provide support for the current model run to the pharmaceutical industry's require-ments. Individual progestins could possibly still be patented and branded and prescribed at individualized levels, but if a woman tested as likely to react adversely to hormonal contraceptives a customer would be lost.

Research scientist Dr Kirsten Oinonen of Lakehead University researched into whether some women are more sensitive to the side effects, particularly emotional and sexual, of oral contraceptives. She writes, "Many women experience emotional or physical side effects when taking oral contraceptives (OCs). Despite the potential impact on women's health and well-being, there are no valid methods to screen women for their risk of OC side effects." The study suggests a possible role for prenatal testosterone exposure and both androgen action and sensitivity in women's experience of OC side effects. The external indicator of testosterone exposure is comparative finger length.

All women will be changed by hormonal contraceptives, but not all women will experience the extreme physical and emotional impacts that they have the potential to provoke. If women could learn that their hormone profile is individual to them, that its peaks and troughs are part of life and that "being hormonal" is more of a neutral statement of the every day experience of every woman (and man for that matter) then they might question the need to medicalize hormonal changes.

If every bodily experience specific to women, pregnancy, menstruation, menopause, is treated as though it were a disease then, as Barbara Seaman once said, it appears that being female is a disease.

Women in today's society are achieving to a high standard and setting standards even higher for themselves. When confronted with their lack of knowledge about their bodies they may feel a sense of embarrassment or even shame. This might exhibit itself as defensiveness. Matus coaches women coming off hormonal contraceptives and finds she must often work with them through this defensiveness from the start. When teaching women about their bodies she often must help women first deal with their sense of shame. Women are taught to separate their bodies from their minds and to consider the body an entity requiring oppression and management. Matus claims that if the body, through its interaction with the drugs they have chosen to take, causes them suffering, and perhaps even loses them a job, a partner, a choice in life, because of that suffering, the woman may see this an yet another indication of her body failing her, or betraying her.

Matus tells her clients that the contraceptive drugs and devices are used to harness the body, but if we don't know how those drugs and devices work then it is not women who are in control, but the drugs and devices. The further women progress in all areas of life and the more equal their standing to men, the more profound the feeling of personal failure when they learn the impact of a choice made from such a complex position.

For every woman who goes online to share her story and actively cites her desire to help other women who may be suffering in silence there are hundreds more who share their story but flagellate themselves. We are too concerned with viewing ourselves as free, self-actualizing agents. To quote Margaret Talbot in the *New Yorker*, paraphrasing Marx, "women make their own circumstances, but not under circumstances of their own making."

Feminism has become synonymous with the word "choice." The current movement has been branded "choice feminism" in the media. A large reproductive rights initiative is titled 'Feminists for Choice.' If feminism is about choice, then are the consequences of the available choices the responsibility of the individual female consumer or the collective? Even if active and self-defined feminists do disagree with the equation between feminism and choice, the mainstream dilution of the feminist message has produced a culture in which many women assume a plethora of choice is the only requirement for true freedom. Contraception conversations center around the questions of why there are not more choices.

The New York Times reported of choice feminism, "This seemingly innocuous term, coined by a lawyer and scholar, Linda R. Hirshman, in the December issue of The American Prospect, refers to the popular feminist philosophy that in her words declares "a woman could work, stay home, have 10 children or one, marry or stay single." "It all counted as 'feminist' as long as she chose it," Ms. Hirshman wrote."

As with many contemporary activist movements the underlying suggestion is that we are capable of buying ourselves out of oppression.

Kissling writes of this emphasis on individualism and autonomy, "The woman who uses Seasonique is a sexual subject in control of her body. Through her choice to take this birth control pill rather than others, she is able to keep her feminine body under easy surveillance and maintain sexual and economic availability to others. With the discipline of cycle-stopping contraceptives, she can maintain a docile body that is not disruptive of the neoliberal economy or neoliberal state—nor is it disruptive of the demands of patriarchy."

We are not buying ourselves out of oppression but into complicit submission.

Kissling refers to Foucault's concept of "docile" bodies. Foucault writes in *Discipline and Punish*, "The human body was entering a machinery of power that explores it, breaks it down and rearranges it. A 'political anatomy', which was also a 'mechanics of power', was being born; it defined how one may have a hold over others' bodies, not only so that they may do what one wishes, but so that they may operate as one wishes, with the techniques, the speed and the efficiency that one determines. Thus discipline produces subjected and practiced bodies, 'docile' bodies."

Hormonal contraceptives are tools for a patriarchal society to have a "hold" over women's bodies and the design of these drugs literally changes how those bodies operate. As Martin explores, suppressing the hormone cycle and specifically menstruation, is connected historically to a drive for efficiency. When female biology is understood as volatile and unpredictable, switching off the centrally volatile element of that biology with drugs or devices produces a controlled, suppressed body with a presumed predictable biology. The theory is that women's bodies can be made more useful through chemical control, the practice, however, is somewhat different.

A docile body is a body compliant to these drugs, and as such compliant to society's restrictions. But newer generation pills have provoked a range of emotional changes in women that have made them far from docile. Women have self-reported the side effect of extreme rage. Yet, this rage is turned on their loved ones rather than the cause of their suffering. It is interesting to consider how hysteria has been understood as an indicator of women reacting to their oppressed position in society. The emotional side effects of hormonal contraceptives are not psychosomatic but women are frequently told by their doctors the side effects are just the result of over-thinking, reading too much on the internet or the excessive stress of our lives.

The docile body in today's society, the docile body that best fits the system, is a body that is racked with anxiety and fear. The least disruptive woman is a woman wrapped up in her own nervous breakdown.

We are not meant to look outside of ourselves when we experience side effects from hormonal contraceptives. The majority of women will continue to doubt their experience even after they have come off hormonal birth control and found that they feel better. Their experience of their own reaction is the key but women are taught to distrust their judgment.

If a woman admits to being made miserable by birth control pills will she be trusted to speak out against them or will she be judged for what are seen as her own personal failings?

The number of "pill refugees," as a *Salon* writer once named them, is ever growing. Where do they stand in a culture that refuses to acknowledge the validity of their experience?

There are already many undersold and underused birth control choices available. However, improvements on non-hormonal contraceptive methods demand consumer pressure. It is here that the consumer can wield some immediate power. The Female Condom Project provided print out requests to take to US pharmacies to ask that they stock their shelves with this recently reinvented contraceptive method, now called the FC2. Whether that consumer power can hold up against the power of pharmaceutical companies to promote their product as the only option remains to be seen.

There have been few developments in condom design in the US and UK until recently. Although the Japanese brands Beyond Seven and Crown are frequently voted the best for feel, experience and safety they usually must be bought online. Many are unaware of these brands because they are not available on store shelves. Two independent condom innovators have come about – Theyfit in the UK and Origami in the US.

Theyfit condoms require the man use measuring materials downloaded from the website to provide width and length statistics before they are provided with practically tailor-made condoms.

Origami condoms are made from silicone and concertinaed. They have a male condom; a female condom and a condom specifically for anal sex are in development and as yet awaiting approval by the FDA. *The New Scientist* reports that silicone is more flexible than latex and more effective at blocking viruses and bacteria. Internal lubrication of Origami condoms means they can be put on faster and "its fluid lining is supposed to mimic the vaginal environment, simulating sex without a condom for a man. Ridges on its surface are meant to enhance the experience, making it double as a sex toy." The team is also experimenting with prevention of "backflow" with a specialized reservoir at the tip.

September 26th is the Bayer-sponsored World Contraception Day. In their promotion of this event they name themselves "world leader in hormonal contraceptives." The event is a branding campaign to push their products on new markets. It's a marketing effort akin to McDonalds sponsoring the London Olympics, an attempt on the part of corporation to appear to have interests beyond increasing profits.

Certain technologies currently in research will require a funding boost if they are ever to come to market. The Duet and SILCs diaphragms are one-size-fits-all and therefore do not require a fitting with a doctor and could be obtained without prescription. New devices are nearly always tested first in developing countries and then considered for developed nations. There is too much of a push behind the injection and long acting hormonal contraceptives for these inventions to be fully developed and tested without direct public advocacy.

In the 1960s and early 1970s in reaction to the continued illegality of abortion, Lorraine Rothman and Carol Downer developed a self-help movement for women's health. The leaders learnt how to instigate an early abortion safely and developed the equipment necessary to do so independent of the mainstream medical industry. Women were encouraged in this movement to learn self-examination techniques and to get to know their bodies and how they change through the month and during pregnancy. Armed with a speculum small groups of women were taught to study the vagina and cervix by looking at other women's and their own. Through this initiative they produced manuals that detailed knowledge of women's bodies far beyond that of a trained gynecologist.

"To us self-help means taking control of our bodies and our health care," Downer is reported as saying in *A Woman's Book of Choices*. Lorraine Rothman added, "What did women do before they had doctors? It can't be that hard. Let's just take back the technology, the tools, the skills, and whatever else we need."

One technique the movement developed was menstrual extraction – used not just for early abortion but also to shorten and lighten a woman's period. Through their methods an entire period's worth of menstrual blood could be removed in a few hours instead of being experienced over a length of days. They saw the possibilities in this for female athletes and for any woman for whom their period was inconvenient at one time or another. A woman cannot do a menstrual extraction alone but needs the help of one or two other women. Menstrual extraction is practiced across the world, often in countries where abortion is illegal. In Cuba menstrual extraction is offered to any woman whose period is two week's late regardless of whether they have taken a pregnancy test. But in the US, the Roe v Wade ruling put to a halt to this underground educational movement.

Downer described her first experience viewing a medical procedure – the insertion of an IUD – "I got a glimpse of her cervix and was completely bowled over. It was such a shock to see how simple and accessible our anatomy is. I realized if women just had some basic information about their bodies, they could take care of themselves."

In a 2012 piece Downer writes that now is the time for women to rediscover menstrual extraction with abortion becoming more expensive, less accessible and more controversial. Downer states that despite recurrent fears she doubts Roe v Wade would ever be reversed. "Why?" she asks, "The hypocritical leaders of this country, both right and left, recognize that the U.S. industrialized economy is built on the small nuclear family with both parents working, so large families are out. This lowers the birth rate, which satisfies the leaders, who, rather than creating a more just, sustainable society, think reducing women's fertility solves social problems such as pollution and poverty. Immigration, legal and illegal, produces the influx of workers and soldiers so desired by the conservatives who have created an unjust society where one percent possess the wealth and resources, further enabling them to keep the 99 percent low-paid and politically powerless."

Downer discusses how the women's liberation movement started out trying to change the whole system, but settled with changing women's status within that system. Women are losing control of their sexual and reproductive lives from demands on the aesthetics of their genitals to radical interventions in their births, but they believe hormonal contraceptives and the innovations of these methods are providing them with control. Downer's cross-country tour for teaching women self-examination came in the wake of the Nelson Pill Hearings.

Downer's on-going project 'Women's Health in Women's Hands' provides information on managing your own fertility. Downer wrote a guide titled *How to Avoid the Gynecologist's Office* and her advice follows this anti-medical establishment and anti-pharmaceuticals sentiment. The female condom, diaphragm, cervical cap and fertility awareness methods are front and center. The network of Feminist Health Centers of California that sprung up as a result of the movement still exists today. They provide in-depth information on the impact of hormonal methods and fertility awareness method training.

The Shodhini Institute is the new incarnation of Downer's collectives. Founded in Indian tradition, the organization provides self-help classes, education on natural remedies for gynecological problems and lessons in the fertility awareness method. The Shodhini Institute asserts its values as "body autonomy," "body attunement and mindfulness" and "guilt free" body exploration.

An internationally distributed zine translated from the French original by Isabelle Gauthier, *Hot Pantz*, is a guide to "do-it-yourself gynecology." Gauthier writes in introduction, "We believe it's integral for women to be aware of and in control of their own bodies. The recipes we present here have been known and practiced for centuries, passed down from mother to daughter, and have survived the censorship of the witch-hunts. Our intent is simple and practical: to help break away from the medical establishment's tentacular grip on our bodies." This photocopied and annotated booklet is packed with information on alternative remedies for the many health issues for which the pill is so often prescribed and can cause from heavy periods to yeast infections to ovarian cysts.

Self-help could be the natural extension of those feelings expressed by many of the women who suffer from the side effects of hormonal contraceptives. Their sense of personal responsibility would become more positive and proactive if it were translated into taking action to become knowledgeable about their bodies. The desire for control and the need to experience our free agency could be harnessed this way. The self-help movement of the past and present has marked out a possible future for the "surveillance" of female bodies - women choosing to monitor themselves in order to have autonomy over their reproductive and sexual lives is an alternative path.

Practicing this as a collective could forge a resistance to our oppressive culture. The comments boards on which women exchange advice regarding coming off hormonal contraceptives show that there is already the potential arena for encouraging women to reconnect with their bodies, their femaleness and each other.

Section Six: The Addiction

"The sick woman was not far off from the ideal woman." Barbara Ehrenreich, *For Her Own Good.*

"My doctor put me on Ortho-Micronor, touting its ability to clear up acne. My skin started to develop a dewy sheen, as if I lived in a perpetual state of afterglow. I enjoyed this new, fresh look and didn't notice anything much different about the rest of my body, except for the fact that I stopped wanting to have sex with my boyfriend. I started to lose weight. Of course I saw this as another unexpected bonus, dropping thirty pounds in the course of a year. What looked near anorexic to other people I interpreted as sexy, young, light. Except I was also losing my hair in large clumps when I showered. I was finding it hard not to feel paranoid almost constantly. I had stopped writing, stopped having any creative thoughts at all. I felt afraid everywhere we went that we would either get in a fatal car accident or be murdered. I was afraid I was exhibiting early signs of schizophrenia and came off. I went back on the pill before getting married. Right away, I felt awful. Not only did I lose my libido again, sex became extremely painful. I have no real memory of those years on the new pill except sort of floating through them, dissociated from both my body and my mind. I decided to go off when I developed break-through bleeding. I feel like I was frozen in time those years I took the pill. I have regained my sexuality and my sanity." - Suzanne

The fix

The mainstream birth control conversation emphasizes that contraceptive choice is a personal issue and as such beyond judgment. In 2012 the campaign 'This Is Personal' came about in response to the furor of the religious Right in the US. "Keep the government out of my uterus" is the message. This standpoint and attitude does not facilitate conversation between women about any of the many problems they may encounter when making these choices. Just as with the 'No Controversy' campaign such projects ostensibly attempt to empower women while actually helping only to silence them.

This third wave feminist approach to reproductive rights isolates women. The collective is not present here and individualism prevails. Sharing information, experiences, knowledge or advice has become a minefield of manipulated meaning. Women are attacked for voicing their discontent with the contraceptive choices offered to them. The standpoint assumes far more independence in the choice making than most women will encounter at their doctor's office. "This subject is between me and my doctor," is the oft-repeated phrase. This elevates the relationship between patient and doctor out of reality.

In response to an article of my own a commenter stated, "Your experiences don't belong in this article as any kind of evidence towards a broader social/medical problem for every girl. The way you make your personal decisions has little to do with anyone else," and, "You've especially avoided facing the realization that your personal experiences have nothing to do with anyone else."

Sanders examined the self-improvement culture in a piece for *Bitch* magazine entitled 'Eat, Pray, Spend.' There is, she argues, an "obsession with wellness." Within this culture enlightenment comes about as a result of finding a good man, a great beauty regime, a yoga body and the life experience that can only come from expensive new-age vacations and retreats.

Wellness could be seen to be connected to the idea of perfection. The underlying narrative of this search for wellness might be reduced to: "Women are inherently and deeply flawed, in need of consistent improvement throughout their lives. Those who do not invest in addressing their flaws are ultimately doomed to make themselves, if not others, miserable."

By taking hormonal contraceptives women are told that they will, in a sense, achieve "wellness." Self-improvement via the pill is part of the wider consumer economy message of self-improvement through spending. Sanders points out that the women writers of "priv-lit" often present themselves as working for their own, very personal and intimate needs when in fact they are acting in response to those needs that are created for them by this culture. These women are not rising above a society that makes them feel "unwell" or faulty for being a woman, but perpetuating the assumption that women are sick and need to be made better. After ingesting the negativity towards femaleness they react in a way that confirms the validity of that negativity.

The culture surrounding the selling of the pill creates a false context in which women are oppressed by the insistence of undefined authorities that they experience their femaleness. This context is made possible by the production of a false image of femaleness that is far divorced from any original. Sanders remarks that when such women discuss being "healthy" that healthy is never an end in itself but only a means to the more desired end of appearing "healthier" and thus more attractive. The desired result of "healthiness" is attracting a man.

Tampons and sanitary towels were originally accessibly only to the rich. They were signifiers of a glamorous lifestyle. It was by no accident that Yasmin and Yaz entered the market as the most expensive birth control pills and then became an essential element of aspirational living. For this current recessionary era we are encouraged to spend carefully on what are termed as "investment pieces." The Chanel handbag of the birth control world is a Mirena IUD or implant. The pay out may be big, but it is a true bargain in the long term.

We must feel there is something missing if we are to go out searching for it. The missing element cannot be a part of all human experience, but only intrinsic to our own life. We must look, seek and search to become whole. We must feel incomplete; we must feel we are not our "true selves" for this sense of lack to be created and for the need to fill the void to arise.

Ehrenreich argues that it was during the 1960s that sex became fully separated from reproduction. The pill's introduction went a long way to help society sever this tie. Once sex and reproduction were no longer connected, it became easier to detach sex from ideas of commitment and affection. Ehrenreich suggests that sex could be simply commodified and sold back to people in the form of all of the 'sexy' consumables and products that might help a person become 'sexy.'

Society favored a nuclear family in which both parents were expected to go to work in order to provide the funds to sustain their lifestyle. Yet Helen Gurley Brown's book *Sex and the Single Girl* set up the single life as the most glamorous choice. Single women who had a string of relationships prior to finding someone to settle down with and marry were viewed as surefire spending machines.

Ehrenreich quotes a marketing company director from an interview conducted in the early 1970s regarding the growing trend towards singledom: "There's nothing in this that business would be opposed to. People living alone need the same things as people living in families. The difference is there's no sharing. So really this trend is good as it means you sell more products. The only trend in living arrangements that business does not look favorably on is this thing with communes, because here you have a number of people using the same products."

As Levy writes, "Making sexiness something quantifiable makes it easier to explain and to market. If you remove the human factor from sex and make it about stuff then you can sell it. Suddenly sex requires shopping."

Ehrenreich explains that as women were accepted into a man's world they were also marginalized. "Human values" were pushed out to make way for the more socially supported traits of selfishness and individualism. The values of contemporary society were hot-housed in the 60s. The profitability of relationships, this drive for self-fulfillment, this culture was settled and solidified.

As not men or women, but rather consumers, we have our maleness and our femaleness manipulated, repackaged and sold back to us. It is more useful that we do not know what it is to be female, that we do not own this knowledge but that we must buy back the knowledge via signifying products piece by piece. The idea of the "real" or "original" in terms of gender is used against us. Even if there is no original femaleness, there is the body. There is a real dichotomy of sickness and wellness and there is the human experience of the body in sickness and in wellness.

This striving for self-perfection is also bigger than gender; it is a resistance to death. Our bodies and their changing and ever aging nature are indicators of our mortality. The way the pill is presented as a miracle cure reflects on the human need to combat aging and defend against inevitable death. The search for enlightenment is in part a search for the meaning in life. Yet, as Faulkner writes *As I Lay Dying*, it is women that are "tied to the earth" and therefore it is toward women and their bodies and biology that this anxiety and fear of death is targeted.

We are all too happy to disregard our biology as women, and our humanity as people. The pill is an interior reflection of exterior conformism through body shape, hair color and appearance. It is an act of homogenization that resists the collective. It is sameness with no understanding of similarity.

The fall-out

In 2007 a study was released that claimed strippers make more money in tips when they are ovulating than during the rest of the month. It claimed they make the least when they are menstruating. Dancers in the study made approximately $70 an hour during their fertile time, $35 while menstruating and $50 otherwise. Strippers taking the pill averaged $37 and those not taking the pill averaged $53.

Psychology Today summarized, "Birth control could lead to many thousands of dollars lost every year."

Research relating to how women change through their cycle is always subject to media vitriol. Studies frequently use only a small group of women and contain other obvious limitations. There is an obvious difficulty in funding studies of this sort that produce results not useful to any pharmaceutical company. There are no drug companies looking to aid researchers in discovering the potential benefits of a woman's natural hormone cycle.

One fair criticism, although never mentioned in media coverage, is that research scientists do not tend to know how to teach women to track and determine their ovulatory period and the women in the studies themselves don't know when they are actually ovulating. The studies likely make a guess based on the woman's previous cycle length. Without being specific about this data results will vary.

If released research confirms that the uterus and ovaries are only useful for pregnancy and that the hormone cycle makes women erratic and irrational then it is happily accepted. If the research says anything that opposes this view women balk at what are assumed to be the misogynistic motivations of the researchers. It is concluded that these scientists must be trying to draw attention to how different women are in order to justify their oppression.

A writer for *Jezebel* introduced a piece on a study that suggested men are drawn to dancing women more so when they are ovulating than when they are in other phases of their cycle with: "In the latest study about how we all might as well still be cave people when it comes to sexual activity."

The researcher of this study stated that, "The findings that estrus impacts earnings could have implications for women selling cars or giving big presentations as C.E.O.s," Miller says. "Should women schedule big job interviews during certain weeks of the month? We don't know. But maybe."

Instead of putting funds into research already underway at CeMCOR into the health benefits of ovulation and the protection consistent ovulatory cycles might provide against heart disease, breast cancer and osteoporosis, funds are used to reduce this vital bodily function to its usefulness in terms of money-making. These studies commodify ovulation as Gray's *The Optimized Woman* might be said to commodify menstruation.

The religious Right unfortunately dominates what discussion there is about the far-reaching effects of widespread use of hormonal contraceptives. The valid question of whether the impact of the pill on an individual woman might reflect consequences for women as a whole is undermined by their repressive agenda.

A group of Roman Catholic Nuns produced a video that extolled the damage done by women using contraception, birth control of any kind although with an emphasis on the most popular methods. The video contains statements that explain simplistically the impact of hormonal birth control on women's attraction to men and vice versa and the effect of synthetic hormones on the environment as well as an explanation of the known side effects. Also included are complaints about women degrading themselves and "killing babies" in the first days of egg fertilization plus suggestions that birth control causes "homosexual behavior." Their conclusion is that contraception is "sinful." The initial valid and what should be thought-provoking points are lost amid senseless noise.

The abstinence-promotion group 1Flesh produced a video that presents common misinformation that is used to explain the impact of the birth control pill. The woman presenter makes the claim that the medical industry desires to "reduce all women to the same manageable cycle." She argues that "nowhere else in the medical world would this approach be considered good medicine." And so again, actual legitimate information about hormonal contraceptives is mixed together with anti-barrier method messages and judgment of women who have sex outside of marriage.

1Flesh proposes that women use the Catholicism-based Creighton Method for avoiding pregnancy. This is a fertility awareness method that requires women monitor the changes to their cervical mucus and temperature to discern when they are fertile. It provided the foundation for Matus' secular Justisse Method, which adds in the charting of cervical position.

Religious methods of natural family planning differ from the secular FAM versions in their communication by the practitioners. As a rule, practitioners will not coach unmarried women or couples. Although the rhythm method, as said, is not effective it does not represent all religious-based methods. The founder of the Creighton Method, Dr Thomas Hilgers, is an endocrinologist whose methodology is correct but presentation is founded in oppressive Catholic teachings regarding women.

NaProTechnology is the method used under Creighton to reestablish women's cycles and fertility by diagnosing and treat underlying issues. The motivation may be to avoid the IVF process, which goes against Catholic teachings, but it is still more in tune with women's bodies.

1Flesh ambitiously envisages a world in which their teachings will reverse the "sky-high rates of divorce, abortion, and STDs" and aid "a world bored with sex and bored with romance" by bringing us their concept of "sex free from fear, love free from use, and a world of people who love and respect their own bodies."

Animosity towards this kind of criticism of contraception, and hormonal contraception in particular, makes an honest discussion difficult. It is not absurd to imagine that if up to fifty percent of women experience negative emotional effects from the pill that this might have a social consequence. It is not bizarre to wonder if the pill's part in detaching women from their bodies has a knock-on impact in how they act and interact.

The pill did not cause women's sexual liberation, women were having sex before marriage and using the diaphragm to do so before the pill was released. The religious Right's assumption is that without contraception – easy and accessible contraception particularly – people would have less sex outside of marriage.

If we come from a point of intelligence and critical analysis we should be able to make assertions about how hormonal contraceptives may have shaped women's experiences. If we accept that all women are changed by use of hormonal contraceptives and that this change impacts their individual life experiences then what does this mean for women as a whole?

With eighty percent of women using the pill at some point in their lives, and twelve million having taken a tablet just today why has this collective experience of a powerful mind and body altering drug not been considered as essential to women's progress? The pill profoundly changes women and yet we have only examined its popularity through the lens of its benefits as a contraceptive.

We could argue for the pill's role in the rise of what Levy terms "raunch culture." Sexuality as performance is a concept that could more easily take hold in women who have had their libidos dampened by drugs. For us, sexuality has to be performance because we have little interest in sex for ourselves. Our own physical responses and thoughts have been subjugated. We act sexy in compensation for not feeling sexy.

A need for heightened stimulation in sex is driven in part by the impact of the pill on women's bodies. Hormonal contraceptives not only diminish libido but also impair sensitivity of all of the senses. We don't know to what extent pill provoked changes in hormone levels as they are related to biological attraction could have on choice of partner, success of relationships or the nature of those relationships. If on an anecdotal level we understand that women leave their partners at a high rate once they choose to come off the pill, what might be the wider effect of such a phenomenon?

The idea of over-compensation through behavior is often discussed in regards to gender dysphoria. A person might behave in a hyper-masculine or hyper-feminine way to compensate for a lack of personal connection to that gender. The person therefore performs to fit into society in a way that best befits the gender they are assigned by others. Hyper-femininity is seen in the trend for plastic surgery that increases breast size, backside size and decreases the size of the waist. We do not feel our bodies are our own.

Blaming birth control for problems both personal and social is as unpopular and controversial as blaming biology has been for decades. This reactionary response is rooted somewhat in how we view the effect of biology on men. That particular discussion draws out fears of threats to the institutions of monogamy, the nuclear family, even civilization, as we know it.

What is the social impact of providing eighty percent of generally healthy women with a drug that makes them sick?

It is a question that mirrors the queries of the many women who, when they come off the pill, ask what their lives might have been without it. They wonder - would they have stayed with that one boyfriend? Taken that year abroad? Got that promotion? Or simply enjoyed more of their experiences?

In *Sex, Time and Power* Leonard Schlain turns this question on the hormone therapy treatments prescribed to women going through menopause. He asks, "Is HRT a Mephistophelian bargain that trades assertiveness and power for youth and beauty? By artificially maintaining high levels of estrogen and/or progesterone, HRT nearly completely negates the benefits that relatively higher testosterone levels might bestow upon a woman...Patriarchy and misogyny overshadow the current structure of human societies and prevent many women from achieving their full potential as leaders. It cannot be known whether or not women would play an even greater role on the world's stage if they were willing to forgo the visible and metabolic benefits they derive from HRT. What would be the result if instead they embraced the power Mother Nature gave them?" He may have the endocrinology science confused, however the provocation is powerful.

Chikako Takeshita in her book *The Biopolitics of the IUD* explores Foucault's concept of biopower through the development of the IUD as a method for reproductive control. Biopower is explained by Takeshita as the need in modern societies to regulate bodies in order to progress. It is indeed a central element of the functioning success of those societies. Pharmaceutical contraceptives control women's bodies, but women have grasped them with both hands in a bid to be liberated from the disciplines of gender and even class. Through medical contraception there is the promise of rising up through the social ranks.

Takeshita philosophically intertwines the colonization of the world with the colonization of women's bodies. She believes women are viewed as an individualized mass. Pharmaceutical birth control is created on the foundational assumption that all women's bodies are the same. The development of the IUD is her perfect illustration. The sizing of the copper IUD was originally created for an imaginary standardized uterus that was created from an average of gathered statistics on uterus sizes. However, in reality the size of women's uteruses varies dramatically.

"Researchers exclusive interest in the uterus displaced women's agency in favor of biology. Homogenizing their bodies further muted their individuality and agencies," writes Takeshita. Prior to the pill's approval it was tested on just 1,600 women, effectively covering 40,000 cycles. A small pool of women from only one community provided results believed to be applicable to all women.

Takeshita cites historian Andrea Tone's description of the IUD as "technological violence inflicted against the female body." There is indirect violence in the lack of consent procured from the poor and the young for whom the IUD has been historically predominantly prescribed and in the refusal to remove by doctors once their patients return to them with complaints. Takeshita also refers to the physical "violence" of inserting a device that must produce a certain level of bodily damage to meet its end. In her examination of the use of the IUD in population control programs she asserts that technologically managed bodies open up new economic markets.

Sandra Bartky explains the result of this disciplinary power wielded through birth control as the production of "docile bodies," which she describes as "ornamental, passive and unthreatening." We must be unthreatening to both progress and the status quo.

The producers of the IUD took advantage of women's concerns over the pill with the tagline "Off the pill...now what?" Hormonal contraceptives are a more efficient way of producing the truly docile body.

Women who physically expelled their IUDs through their vaginas in the early days of the device's development were classed as having "angry uteruses" or putting up a "uterine protest." This problem was framed as the uterus attacking the device and as an "active battle between the developer's devices and women's bodies."

Such war terminology and practice might be applied to the predicament of those women who when they complain of side effects from the pill are counter-attacked with long acting methods that make it harder for them to resist control by synthetic hormones.

The pharmaceutical companies, the doctors, society as a whole backs women's compliance to drugs and devices. The history of the IUD reveals the shift in methodology from "coercion" in regards to women in developing countries and those living below the poverty line in developed countries to "convenience" for the middle class women of the Western world. Prior to the Affordable Care Act Bayer provided free Mirenas to the uninsured under an affiliated health program.

Takeshita writes that drug inserts allow women to conform to the requirements and standards of a market that forced her to be "a willing and legally (if not physically) safe consumer."

Section Seven: The Recovery

"If a woman loves her own body, she doesn't grudge what other women do with theirs. If she loves femaleness she champions its rights," Naomi Wolf, *The Beauty Myth*.

"Since the age of sixteen I've been on many different kinds of pill, had the contraceptive injection and the non-hormonal IUD, all with very different, very unpleasant side effects. I've been on Microgynon, Femodene, Yasmin, Cilest, Ovrette and Loestrin. Symptoms have ranged from significant increase in breast size, severe painful mouth ulcers, loss of sex drive, significant increase in appetite leading to weight gain, monthly bouts of thrush, depression, fits of rage, fatigue, suicidal thoughts and loss of focus and motivation. Last year I thought I'd try the pill again, after one week of being on Cilest I fell into a deep depression and wanted to kill myself." – Rebecca

Withdrawal

With a lack of support and only the message "stay on the pill" at every turn, women find that even when they do decide to stop taking hormonal contraceptives they are soon scared back to them. Fear of pregnancy, the withdrawal symptoms or just the experience of the strangeness and unfamiliarity of the return of their own cycle can make the transition a struggle.

In collaboration with Wershler I produced a guide to ditching the pill in the hope of providing a breadth of information available in one easily digestible article for those women otherwise relying solely on the testimonies and advice of online commentators. We frame the abandonment of pharmaceutical contraceptives as a rebellion against the establishment's attempt to control women's bodies. The piece is heavily hyperlinked to sources and resources.

The introduction reads - "Throw out your pills, rip off your patch, pull out your ring and take back control. There is more to birth control than prescription medications. This act of rebellion won't be easy, and it won't be for everyone. But if you're mad as hell and not willing to take it anymore, here's a primer on how it can be done."

My experience of withdrawing from the pill truly opened my eyes to my complicated involvement with this drug. It was then that realized I had become addicted to the pill. I kept a couple of packets of Femodette for months and there wasn't a morning I didn't consider taking it again. I had no idea how my body would feel naturally or what it would do naturally. As I was enthusiastically telling everyone I knew what I'd read about the side effects of the pill before I had accepted this information for myself. I thought how good it would have been to write through my experience with Yasmin. Describing going through my worst times with that drug and documenting my realization that other women were going through this too would have been valuable reading, but then I would have needed motivation, energy and initiative to have even considered that.

Within days of stopping taking the pill "for good" as I saw it, I panicked over using condoms alone and the ensuing worry caused me to rush to a clinic for the emergency pill. In the following week I felt as though I might be pregnant as the withdrawal coupled with the Plan B produced nausea, a strange metallic taste in the back of my mouth, bleeding and cramps. By the end of that week I was convinced I was having a baby. Even though I'd sworn off birth control pills I soon reached for another drug to make my anxiety, and the developing fetus as I saw it, go away.

One moment I would be asking - why are women still taking these drugs? The next I was feeling desperate and pondering whether the pill was the answer to all of my problems, old and new.

A few weeks later, I noticed that my senses were becoming more acute. Food tasted better and my touch was more sensitive. I'd stopped feeling achingly tired by eight o'clock each night. My brain fog cleared and this allowed me to think read and concentrate without coming up against the blocks I'd had for so long. The withdrawal produced a low humming sense of dread similar to that I experienced under Yasmin, but once that lifted I felt more grounded than I could remember being before. I wanted to see where this would progress and making my experience public through the blog bolstered me in the resolve to stick with my decision. That said, I still found it hard to trust the condoms which I used in conjunction with spermicide, even though I'd read so much that undermined that unfounded distrust.

I first knew when I was ovulating because I experienced a dull pain in my side in the middle of my cycle that would last for several hours.

My skin and hair took a turn for the worse and I can admit I found this perhaps the hardest part of the transition. It was this that made me question my decision. I had a tough time dealing with the acne that was worse than I recalled ever having as a teenager. The greasy, limp hair was a depressing morning welcome. I thought about the many women who must get to this point and turn back, figuring as you might that either they have "naturally" bad skin and greasy hair which the pill "cured" or just that the pill was the only efficient way to keep this under control.

I saw the pill's power firsthand by seeing what happened when it was taken away.

It's difficult to express how depressing it is to experience acne in your late twenties without sounding pathetic, but I believe the resurgence of hormones that causes this when coming off the pill, along with the perhaps permanent hormone imbalances it produces are a integral reason women find it hard to ditch hormonal contraceptives despite side effects.

It became a battle between my new naturally rooted emotions and the symptoms of withdrawal that affected my mood. On some pill brands and at some points in the last ten years I had felt flat and indifferent. Although I did experience deep lows and anxiety for some years, it was my ability to feel truly excited, happy, content or blissful that had completely disappeared.

It took me a couple of weeks to realize the withdrawal I was going through was in fact a drug withdrawal. I noticed the insomnia first and put it down to changing work shifts, too much television before bed – anything I could think of but the withdrawal. I had two big meltdowns of the like I hadn't seen since in the haze of Yasmin but I still wasn't certain what was happening to me. When I got stressed it was like a quicksand of emotions. I could not see the wider perspective, but only a big black hole of despair.

I had, of course, the nagging worry that this withdrawal would not pass. I would read online accounts from women that said it had been two months, six months, even two years before they felt better. Some said that after a few years they still had some issues.

As the pill left my system, I knew I would be "responsible" for my moods. It had taken me so long to realize that my anxiety was provoked by the pill, but then I had to worry I would eventually find out my problems were deeper, unsolvable, just me.

It was a co-dependent relationship. I was left wondering who I might be and I was scared to carry on without the pill and find out. I hadn't been without it since I was seventeen.

Three months off the pill and I felt brighter but still disorientated. I felt as though I were relearning how to react and interact. My spectrum of feelings in their depth and intensity were overwhelming – no longer was it just flatness or a freak out. I had a fullness of feeling coming through a haze of chemicals.

It was about this time that I started researching into the

fertility awareness method as a way to support my change to non-hormonal contraceptives.

Wershler used fertility awareness as her method of birth control for twenty-five years. She has written extensively about how there is a profound lack of support from the medical industry and society at large for women who choose not to use hormonal contraceptives, for any reason. She believes that the gap in information created by the refusal to acknowledge women who don't want to use a drug or device contributes to the unplanned pregnancy rate. Wershler also believes this standpoint shows a lack of respect for women's health and their agency.

The importance of what she coined "body literacy," a term she describes as "learning to observe, chart and interpret our menstrual cycle events...a life skill that helps us understand how our sexual, reproductive and general health and well-being are connected to our menstrual cycles. Body literacy supports, if not compels, our fully informed participation in health-care decision making."

In our collaborative guide for women seeking non-hormonal alternatives Wershler writes, "Fertility awareness, like riding a bicycle, is a life skill. If you can knit a sweater, read a balance sheet, or master French cooking and Adobe InDesign, you can learn to observe, chart and interpret your menstrual cycle events. Referred to as natural birth control, the secular Fertility Awareness Method (FAM), and its religious-based counterpart Natural Family Planning (NFP), are based on observing and interpreting scientifically proven signs of fertility to prevent or achieve pregnancy and monitor your reproductive health. FAM is absolutely not the same thing as the ineffective Rhythm Method, which tries to predict fertility based on the length of past cycles. Don't believe those who tell you that FAM doesn't work; women using it can achieve effectiveness rates as high as the pill – 99.4 percent. But unlike Catholic NFP, FAM is pro-choice and incorporates barrier methods, emergency contraception and abortion. If you're single you should know that using the fertility awareness method in conjunction with condoms with added spermicide even during your fertile phase has been shown to be 98.2% effective at preventing pregnancy – so it's just as suitable for the one-night stand as the committed relationship."

A comprehensive study of nine hundred women over a ten-year period conducted by research scientists at the University of Heidelberg in Germany found that FAM has a very high effectiveness rate – with 99.4% effectiveness with abstinence during fertile window and 98.2% effectiveness using barriers during this time.

In an article published in the *Journal of the American Board of Family Medicine* writers Dr Stephen R. Pallone and Dr George R. Bergus state, "modern FAMs have typical-use unintended pregnancy rates of 1% to 3% in both industrialized and nonindustrialized nations." They report that frequently doctors have very little knowledge of this method of contraception, however with the fertility awareness method explained to them briefly "more than one in five" women expressed an interest in learning. One to three percent of women use the method in the US currently, "Despite an improved understanding of the science underlying FAMs, rates of use have declined to 11% from 22% of married couples in 1955." The piece concludes with a recommendation that doctors offer the method as a "reasonable choice" for pregnancy prevention and that interested women are provided with information and referred to a certified provider.

Chris Evans, a locum SHO in emergency medicine, argues in a letter to the *British Medical Journal* that the Guttmacher Institute and United Nations Population Fund have a bias towards what is termed "modern" contraception and incorrectly suggest alternative methods of contraception like FAM are "much more likely to fail." He states, "The pill, male condoms, female condoms, and spermicides are all classified as modern contraception, but their typical use failure rates are 8%, 15%, 21%, and a staggering 29%, respectively. Contrast this with the typical use failure rate of modern methods of natural family planning, such as the Creighton, Billings, and symptothermal methods, which some studies report as around 3%, similar to Depo Provera. In fact, the perfect use failure rates of these methods have been reported as 0.5%, 0.5%, and 0.3%, respectively, comparable to those of the pill, female sterilisation, and the copper intrauterine device."

I was first introduced to FAM by a friend when I was in withdrawal from the pill. She had abandoned hormonal contraceptives due on side effects, specifically the impact on her creativity as she is a writer, and she was using condoms, spermicide and the fertility awareness method together. She avoided penetrative sex during her fertile period. She explained to me how our body temperature changes through the month depending on our hormone cycle.

It was the first time I had heard this, the first time I realized there were times when I was not fertile at all and unable to get pregnant.

It was obvious that it would be extremely helpful to women coming off the pill to have an understanding of their cycles. I could see how beneficial it would be to feel connected to those changes instead of frightened and perplexed. My hormone cycle would be something I was doing, rather than something happening to me. I knew I would feel less anxious about being off the pill if I knew when I was fertile and could interpret my body's signals to know that I was not pregnant.

If I knew when I was fertile I'd be able to stop worrying about being off the pill.

The fertility awareness method with abstinence from penetrative sex during the fertile time is differentiated in teaching from the fertility awareness method with use of condoms when fertile. This is because when using condoms during the fertile window the couple is relying on the effectiveness of the barrier method. Condoms when used in conjunction with a spermicide is a method with 95.65 percent typical use effectiveness rate. Condoms alone have an eighty-five percent effectiveness rate with typical, not perfect use. That said, if you know you are fertile you may be more careful with your condom use and if the condom breaks and you know you're not fertile, you would be saved from taking unnecessary morning-after pills.

At that time I received The Natural Fertility Management kit from Jane Bennett, replete with thermometer, and coincidentally I was reading the "gurlesque" novel *Wetlands* by Charlotte Roche. Written from the point of view of an eighteen year-old woman who is fascinated by her bodily functions, the novel is essentially a series of first person descriptions of her secretions, toilet habits, sex acts and physical explorations and experimentations. These two books complemented each other as they met somewhere in the middle at the exploration of cervical mucus textures. Reading about the protagonist Helen's delight in being human and alive, her lack of shame about her body, reading descriptions of her creating impromptu tampons from toilet paper, made me see the funny side of my own prudishness and anxiety. It wore away at my resistance to getting more intimate with how my body worked.

The religious Natural Family Planning groups encourage abstinence until marriage and then abstinence during fertile times and teach married couples along those lines. Secular FAM teachers will suggest the use of barriers during the fertile phase, or the practice of alternatives to non-penetrative sex. Many women actually find that their libido peaks during ovulation so emphasis on alternatives to penetrative sex during this time may allow them to capitalize on this shift. There are women who feel it is not solely through penetrative sex that they gain the most enjoyment.

Although it is very beneficial to be able to chart your cycle through the month and know your fertile time precisely, just a little body literacy can go a long way. Just knowing that we are fertile for only a few days per month is an important step towards body and self-confidence. Knowing that our hormones fluctuate and experientially understanding the monthly repeated patterns of change to your energy levels and mood can have a very freeing effect. This little information is especially useful to someone who has come off hormonal contraceptives. Such facts are not widely taught or known.

Pati Garcia, co-founder of the Shodhini Institute in Los Angeles, runs self-examination classes for groups of women. She introduces fertility awareness via observation of the cervix over a four-week period. During a cervical self-examination, Garcia asks that women examine and feel between their fingers their cervical mucus. She teaches how the texture of that mucus changes throughout the month and how this signifies fertility.

"I want women to learn first on a visceral level about when they are fertile," Garcia explains.

Garcia has seen an increase in interest in self-help healthcare in the last year. The reasons, she feels, are many and varied: "Women are not being treated with respect by Planned Parenthood or by their doctors. Their questions are not being answered. They are learning that they are their own experts when it comes to their body. They want tools to help them understand."

Garcia believes that women are not presented with non-hormonal options and their right to access, even after they are sick from hormonal birth control, is systematically denied. Without readily available information on non-hormonal methods she questions the validity of women's informed consent. Garcia is convinced that if women had full knowledge of fertility awareness at their disposal, information on how hormonal contraceptives affect the body and understanding of the effective alternatives then they would not to use hormonal contraceptives with such frequency.

The Shodhini Institute encourages open discussion amongst women about their bodies equally to the individual learning process. The open discussion can develop solidarity, unity, compassion and a sense of collective experience. Each woman's body is examined, both by her and the teaching group, and revealed to be different and unique.

The medical establishment's power over women's bodies is overthrown. The image of women, speculums inside vaginas, investigating each other's cervixes is in direct opposition to our mainstream and normalized experience of a doctor staring into a vagina and telling the woman, who has never seen what the doctor is seeing, what is wrong with her body.

My own attempt to find an alternative to the pill was not driven by a need to avoid condoms so it was obvious for me to just add a spermicide. It was at first difficult to track down spermicides in local pharmacies, especially in the small town where I lived at that time.

I knew chemical-based spermicides could be harmful so I looked into natural alternatives but shipping in the Canadian-made Contragel proved expensive. I found out about clinical testing for a new gel, Amphora, which supposedly holds less of a risk of causing UTIs and infections. When I spoke with the Amphora representative about becoming a test subject I said I would be using Amphora or the comparative brand Contragel along with the fertility awareness method. Despite the main objective of the study being to discover the gel's rate of effectiveness at preventing pregnancy, the representative said that as long as I wasn't using another "physical" form of contraception I could be involved.

It was clear that she either did not know how the method works or that she knew but believed its effectiveness would be minimal. We can see from this how a lack of understanding of the fertility awareness method and the continued suppression of this knowledge might have a wide and dramatic impact on contraceptive development as a whole.

Justisse-Healthworks for Women provides training for those wanting to learn how to educate women in fertility awareness as well as providing education for women who want to discover fertility awareness through these tutors and the organization's guides. The Justisse Method is what is called a Sympto-Thermal method of fertility awareness in that it teaches women how to observe, chart and interpret their three main signs of fertility – cervical mucus, cervical changes and basal body temperature shift.

Matus and Justisse Educator Megan Lalonde, produced the guide *Coming off the Pill, the Patch, the Shot and other Hormonal Contraceptives* to help women through the process of coming off the pill and other hormonal contraceptives. They liken the hormonal state of being on the pill to the state of menopause, a comparison they say is "supported by the common physiological changes which are observed in women in menopause and using hormonal contraceptives – infertility, increased risk for breast cancer, cardio-vascular disease, stroke, insulin resistance, bone loss, immuno-suppression, and problematic mood disruption."

The book advises women to chart their coming off the pill cycles to be able to track a return to healthy cycles or to identify specific problem cycles. Additionally the guide outlines a regimen for healthy transition involving the removal of non-nutritional foods, replacement of lost nutrients with supplements, and development of healthy eating habits. As a last resort, bio-identical hormone replacement therapy is suggested to restore the ovulatory and menstrual cycle.

A writer for *No More Dirty Looks*, an online community dedicated to natural and organic cosmetics, writes about her experience on and off the pill, "The best way I can put it is, I sort of felt like a prisoner in my own body...I went off the pill, my skin freaked out...my period went away for the better part of a year."

Blog writer Siobhan introduces an enquiry from a reader who has been through a similar experience. This reader tried to go off the pill but could not carry on without it. She explains that she is trying once again and says, "I accept that my body is going to go on a roller coaster ride. I'm ready for the acne this time. Last time I thought I could just stop taking the pill and my skin wouldn't talk to me. How oily my scalp got and the abundance of acne caught me by surprise. I froze up and caved in and took the pill again. This time, I will be ready for them, and hope to have better ways to deal with them or even prevent them." She finishes her letter with a plea for advice from the community.

Lyndsey Holder writes for xoJane 'My (Mirena) IUD Nearly Ruined My Life.' She describes, "Around the time I had my IUD implanted I began having massive, vomit-inducing panic attacks. I would stay in my bed for days and missed so much work." Holder explains that her breakdown was so severe she checked herself into a rehabilitation center. When she returned she was somewhat better, but still with the device, and it was her husband who suggested that her issues only began once she had the Mirena inserted. She had it removed, "After a full month of having the IUD out of my system, my anxiety was completely under control and I was back to my normal, pre-IUD self. A co-worker was curious why I had missed three months of work the previous year followed by two months of work early in this year. I told her my story and explained about the IUD. She looked back at me in awe. "The same thing happened to me," she said. She became severely depressed and had suicidal ideation. Then she had the IUD removed and she immediately returned to her pre-IUD happy, productive self."

Women often cite their partners as the catalyst for their decision. Their encouragement to stop using a method can play an important role in a woman's choice to move on to natural alternatives.

Whitney Peoples is a student at Emory University writing her thesis on how the public discussions of birth control can shape the choices that women make. She suggests that it is the pharmaceutical industry that shapes this conversation. Women often choose the method that they have seen advertised on TV or in magazines, or they choose the method their friends recommend who have themselves been influenced by commercials.

It is only when women go through the experience of side effects, particularly from those drugs most heavily advertised, that an alternative conversation emerges.

Peoples notes however that these discussions are quickly discredited. The counter-argument is that the majority of women reporting their stories online will have had bad experiences because this is what provokes them to go online in the first place, looking for advice and that therefore they do not represent the totality of experience. Thousands of women are nothing in comparison to the vast numbers that must be happy and without complaint. Peoples highlights how the refutations are founded in pseudo-scientific theories of the menstrual cycle as unhealthy and unnecessary. She sees this as emblematic of how women are unaware of their history and as a consequence repeat messages that originate in misogynistic principles and teachings without realizing.

Of course, if we agree that every woman's body is unique in its hormonal cycle and so every woman will respond differently, this allows for the dismissal of one woman's experience as relevant only to her. Published testimonies are introduced with disclaimers that establish the story as "anecdotal" and therefore not intended to provide medically based insight or advice. These disclaimers are a reaction against those that tear down any criticism of hormonal birth control as irresponsible and misinformed. Yet the disclaimers immediately undermine the woman's experience.

The message is that an experience that is merely personal cannot be political and a woman who is not a doctor or scientist cannot attain knowledge that would support and legitimize her story. Understanding hormonal contraceptives is off-limits to the population that takes them and has no medical background. It is required that every statement be proceeded by "in my experience" even as evidence builds that many women have very similar experiences.

Women's testimonies are restricted in the public space, but a sense of collectivity and community struggles through in the right circumstances. At *No More Dirty Looks* the writer is met with a support and solidarity if not political intent.

The change

Our standpoint on the pill is inextricably linked to our feelings about menstruation. Menstruation activism is illustrative of a movement of resistance against the suppression of periods via hormonal contraceptives. Bobel countered, "I think our only hope of resisting these messages and slowing down if not stopping this body hating is to develop body literacy."

Bobel divides menstrual activists into two groups with differing outlooks. Feminist spiritualist menstruation activists celebrate the exceptionalism of womanhood and thus menstruation. Radical menstruation activists believe women should be able to decide individually how they feel about their period. Many activists from this second group are non-heterosexual identifying. They have created the term "menstruators" to be inclusive of trans-men.

Bobel asserts that it is difficult to "authentically" decide how you personally think or feel about anything without access to comprehensive information. Body literacy provides the possibility of knowing about our bodies and the foundation from which to develop thoughts about our experiences of our bodies. The culture of menstrual shame and secrecy is so ingrained and pervasive it is difficult for anyone to untangle their own views from those opinions absorbed by osmosis.

"Menstrual cycle researchers think of the menstrual cycle as the fifth vital sign, but how many woman grasp how the menstrual cycle functions and how it's related to more than the shedding of the uterine lining? Big Pharma breezes right into this knowledge void. As the beauty industry feeds on insecurity, the menstrual care industry feeds on ignorance and shame," Bobel states.

What women are kept from knowing about menstruation prevents them from understanding ovulation and their own fertility. Bobel hopes we don't judge our own or each other's failings to attain this information, but instead turn to the real culprit behind our ignorance, the medical-industrial complex within a capitalist society.

In an article titled 'In Defense of Hating My Period' Bobel unpacks the polarization of menstruation discussion that alienates women and prevents them from exploring their feelings. She subverts "the pervasive assumption that thinking differently about our cycles necessarily points to loving our cycles." She argues that there is more than just the "two choices on the menstrual menu: I'll have the Obsolete Shaming Nuisance or My Cycle is Womb-alicious." There is a large gray area between loving periods and hating them and ignoring this would be detrimental to efforts to educate about cycles.

Collective action does not require that women are experiencing a collective, hegemonic experience. If we do away with this binary and stop contrasting our own reactions against the reactions of others we can be open and honest without becoming alienated from each other.

I had terribly painful periods as a teenager that made me faint. I spent time on a strong pain-relieving drug called

Feminax, also made by Bayer, incidentally. I secretly enjoyed not having to play sports or go to gym class for five days a month. It felt like my small resistance to the school system. It is easy to assume that once off the pill the heavy periods will return and this is something I feared. I, however, ended up with regular and relatively painless periods.

If I consciously stop pushing myself to work or be productive for the two main days of my period I find my experience is vastly improved. If I deliberately decide to stop trying to achieve too much at this time then I relax and can reach a level of contentment and almost meditative calm that I do not have access to any other time of the month. I am, anyway, intolerant of any pressures on me to do anything I don't enjoy or personally choose to do. I feel I am my most honest during this time and the most judgmental about my own choices. I goad myself to do better. I expect everyone else to be better.

The DIY movement incorporated sanitary products by creating re-usable pads that are now sold commercially as well as through Etsy, for those not interested in making their own. The Diva Cup is an increasingly popular alternative to tampons.

The success of this side of the resistance to period suppression was ignited by environmental awareness. The waste produced and the chemical content of the mainstream products caused women to question the corporate solution to their "women's problems." However growing interest in these alternatives has not yet translated into body acceptance or body literacy.

Pill refugees

Clinical herbalist and founder of the CommonWealth Center for Herbal Medicine, Katja Swift, chronicled her transition off the Mirena after years on the pill and hormonal IUD in a series of articles for *Plant Health* magazine.

Swift believes that traditional healing methods and modern

medicine can complement each other. Even as someone with a background in alternative medicine with a critical eye on the pharmaceutical industry, Swift found the decision to have the Mirena removed very difficult, "I was so afraid to just trust my body, I was so afraid to trust my own healing process. I was so personally and culturally needful of control in this situation." After several months of fertility charting Swift took up using a combination of fertility awareness and condoms for contraception.

Through Swift's experience of the transition she began to question her desire to be "available" at all times, which she saw as the root of her reluctance to give up the IUD. In the article she likens herself when on hormonal contraception to a "24 hour 7/11" always open for business. She began to realize that her period was a time when she naturally wanted to withdraw from her social, work and domestic duties and also from her partner but slowing her productivity during this time made her feel too much guilt and failure.

Swift could see that she needed three days to resist the demands made of her and when she did resist she felt the benefits of taking this stand. She translates this to be the situation of all women, and indeed men. The demands of the contemporary society require that successful participants be available, open and productive at a continuous, unchanging level. As members of this society we have expectations of ourselves to meet these demands and we expect others to provide for us without interruption.

Swift writes, "We expect that our workers will produce the same type of work in July and December. We expect that the things we want to eat and purchase will be available in all seasons. But all these things have cycles and coming back into observance of these cycles is what brings us back to our connection with Earth. Imagine if our society allowed, every month, three days for everyone to stop their daily lives and focus simply on meditation and spiritual work."

Swift writes about quitting hormonal contraceptives as a de facto form of resistance and protest. The misunderstanding and astonishment she came up against when explaining her decision to others revealed to her how unprepared our society is for a woman uninterested in hormonal drugs and devices.

She advises, "Be prepared to fight. You may need to stand up for what you want. Planned Parenthood and other organizations cannot be expected to be supportive of women choosing to cease hormonal birth control (unless they are trying to get pregnant). Friends and partners may question your decision. Be clear about your reasoning, your emotions, and your intent, and you will be able to persist peacefully."

Swift had her Mirena fitted and removed at a Planned Parenthood clinic and came up against difficulties. Planned Parenthood is the pariah of the religious right, and consequently the saint of the liberal left. The organization provides essential care for women at low-cost and this is vital within a for-profit healthcare system, however it has a bias toward hormonal methods of contraception founded on a main motive of pregnancy prevention and population control, which takes precedent over women's health and well-being.

Women confronted with pressure from Planned Parenthood to use a method they don't want find it hard to criticize the organization publicly and this blocks honest discussion about the obstacles women face in making these choices.

The promotion of long-acting methods has deliberately taken advantage of the swelling discontent with the birth control pill. In a NuvaRing television campaign two women at the gym share their weekend stories and one tells the other that her pill packet fell out of her purse whilst she was at a party. She was, it is understood, mortified by this. The friend sympathizes with the assumed embarrassing situation and suggests that she try the more discreet NuvaRing instead.

A widely publicized study presented at the annual American Public Health Association meeting claimed that women who are stressed and depressed are less likely to use birth control pills consistently. Lead researcher Dr Kelli Stidham Hall voiced her concern that an ensuing unwanted pregnancy would worsen such "symptoms." Hall suggests that women suffering from emotional problems should be provided with a long-acting method as a solution as they would not require that they are responsible for remembering to take a pill to secure their infertility. Of the women studied twenty-five percent apparently displayed depression and twenty-five percent had stress symptoms.

Prominent political women's health websites shared this information and none considered that the birth control pill could have been the cause of the stress and depression despite evidence, both scientific and anecdotal, to suggest these side effects are prevalent. Studies into compliance are always going to conclude that compliance can be increased by the avoidance of "user failure" alone.

Dr Hall believes emotional issues are almost always present prior to the pill and this causes women to "perceive" side effects where there are none. Long-acting contraceptive devices are therefore the cure for this perception problem. It is an illustration of how the medical industry will tie itself in knots of contradiction to keep women on hormonal contraceptives. Instead of acknowledging the side effects an intricate system of manufactured choice has been created and at every turn there is a medical treatment for the disease of being young, female and fertile.

Women, especially those in their teens and twenties, are, as *Guardian* writer Kira Cochrane describes, depicted in the media as "insensible, incompetent, insatiable, and intoxicated." The answer to the "ladette," as she is known in the UK, is the LARC. Cochrane remarks that this belief was one of the major social narratives of the noughties decade. Young women are perceived to be having a lot of sex and much of it when intoxicated. The tabloid stories of women behaving "like men" whip up distrust and suspicion. By this logic unwanted pregnancies and abortions are necessarily the result of rampant irresponsibility.

Methods like the Mirena and the implant are seen as the technological fix for a social problem. It helps that these devices are viewed as fantastic gadgetry and, despite being only reconfigurations on old scientific discoveries, can be rebranded as "the future" of contraception. We are supposed to be awed by such advances of science and in this state of wonder unquestioning of the consequences.

We don't know how the pill works, so when the pill is reconfigured into an implant that gap of ignorance is widened and validated.

Evgeny Morozov effectively criticized this TED-promoted culture that celebrates the technological fix for every social ill for the *New Review*. It is a culture he calls "techno-humanitarian."

He writes, "Given TED's disproportionate influence on a certain level of the global debate, it follows that the public at large also becomes more approving of technological solutions to problems that are not technological but political. Problems of climate change become problems of making production more efficient or finding ways to colonize other planets—not of reaching political agreement on how to limit production or consume in a more sustainable fashion. Problems of health care become problems of inadequate self-monitoring and data-sharing."

The "social ill" of women's fertility and subsequent unwanted pregnancies is simplified. Rather than exploring why women have contraceptive failures or choose not to use contraception the problem is "fixed" with a gadget.

The post-human future Ray Kurzweil writes about in *The Singularity is Near: When Humans Transcend Biology* is already here. Women accept techno-evolution in the form of technological adaptations for their bodies. But unlike a steel hip replacement or a bionic arm, these adaptations have a systematic effect of physical and psychological change and do not ensure better health or longevity.

Until very recently the fertility awareness method was primarily taught and learned using the old-fashioned tools of pen and paper. Women chart their temperature, cervical mucus, cervix position and other changes in their general health from month to month on gridded sheets of paper. The most technologically advanced equipment used is the thermometer. Although the method can be self-taught from books, women have been encouraged to seek out trained practitioners and undergo one-to-one training or group training in-person or via an online seminar to achieve the most success and get help with complex cycles.

However, with the advent of the phone app several programs are now available that allow women to enter their gathered information into an app that produces the charts. Most of the apps tell women their fertile and infertile days based on that information.

Kindara is the most sophisticated and comprehensive of these apps. Katie Bicknell and her husband Will Sacks produced the free program with which women can enter their daily statistics – temperature, cervical mucus texture, if and when they have sex, and any additional notes regarding general health and possible mitigating influences and generate a readable chart for interpretation. During the research phase the couple decided to market the app to women who are trying to get pregnant. In promotional copy they only note pregnancy prevention as a possible additional benefit. This was a calculated response to what they saw as pushback for presenting FAM as a contraceptive option. Bicknell believes that the main obstacles to acceptance of fertility awareness are its "image problem" or lack of "brand" recognition coupled with its inconvenient method for delivery and use. They desire to bring FAM into the mainstream and make it as accessible as possible to as many women as possible.

Lauren Bacon, a Kindara user and advisor to the company, remarks, "Most women do not know that ovulation doesn't necessarily happen on day fourteen of your cycle. They don't know an egg can only live for twenty-four hours or that spearm lives for three to five days. They don't know how to identify when they're fertile. Sure it's a process and a bit more effort than taking a pill every day, but in the same way it's harder to learn to eat healthy than having a TV dinner each night. I was on the pill for ten years and I'd thought I was really in charge of my health and my sexuality. I thought I was taking care of myself, but I was missing key information that had been withheld from me." Bacon has been successfully charting for twelve years with one planned pregnancy.

Kindara fits in with the Quantified Self movement as led by editors of *Wired* magazine. The movement pits the individual as the expert of his or her own health against the medical system. Women have tracked their periods for generations and so this is arguably the origin of such self-monitoring. Aside from the benefits to each woman in tracking her cycle, the possibilities of aggregating the statistics of vast numbers of women over many years and learning from that information could be momentous. Funding and resources act as a barrier for those such as Dr Prior of CeMCOR to developing their research. It is very expensive to conduct research that involves a large number of women over a long period of time, but it might be possible to use data from a cross-section of those already tracking their cycles with this technology for research purposes.

An aggregator organization, Cure Together, holds the potential to provide information on individual's differing reactions to the same medications. Self-monitoring is the way most women come to understand they are experiencing the negative effects of hormonal contraceptives. Cure Together provides a space for people to share symptoms, treatments and the side effects of those treatments. Although it could provide an arena for policing the pharmaceutical industry it could also be exploited by those looking for previously unseen gaps to fill with new drugs. Some see this movement as an evolution of biomedicalization and potentially dangerous at a time when a state of good health is viewed as an opportunity for medical intervention as much as illness.

Sharing information about our menstrual cycles could, of course, open women up to judgment and oppressive action and history certainly warns of this potential. A corporation in Norway demanded its female employees wear red bracelets during their periods to provide a visible justification for their, supposedly, more frequent bathroom breaks. The women said they found this "humiliating." German supermarket chain Lidl tried to impose the rule that women in their Czech and Polish stores wear armbands to ensure justification for taking extra breaks. The message behind this action is that menstruation decreases productivity.

The women are not being punished, only expected to provide an excuse for the time not spent at their position. We can speculate that a man with IBS would perhaps have to provide a note from his doctor. The rule encourages certain behavior without explicit requirement. A woman with regular, shorter periods would be judged favorably over a woman with heavier, longer periods. A woman who does not menstruate because she is using hormonal contraceptives would not be judged at all alongside the other female employees. The menstruating women are not afforded any real comforts or understanding, they are only given more breaks in which they are expected to attend to the social duty of hiding the period.

It is interesting that the corporations did not think the women would lie about when they had their period, or perhaps it was assumed it would be somehow too obvious to lie about. An online study of 1,000 women discovered that thirty-eight percent of them admitted to lying about having their period as an "excuse" to not take part in certain activities and events. They said they were most likely to want to avoid sports, exercise or sex. However, the research was sponsored by GlaxoSmithKiline and their pain medication Panadol. These women are in a sense subverting the belief that menstruation is incapacitating for their own use and benefit.

In her work Martin highlights that the bathroom breaks afforded to women provide a space in which they can speak privately away from men. Bathroom breaks can be an opportunity for women to establish their identity, connection, and collectivity. The ostensible requirement of the corporate leaders to increase productivity may hide a desire to limit the amount of unmonitored private time available for all employees.

Even the most ostensibly compassionate corporate practices, such as Google's in-office gym, nap rooms and subsidized meals, that make office life more bearable also encourage longer working hours and total immersion in the work. The aim is to increase productivity. The office space is made so comfortable that employees are not supposed to want to leave.

Would sharing information about our diets, exercise and other habits for public scrutiny provoke us to be better and if so in what ways? As people, workers or consumers?

The Quantified Self movement originally emphasized the possibility for self-experimentation. By tweaking supplements, exercise regimes and diets we might figure out exactly how to enhance our own personal productivity. Employers already police potential and current employees private lives (albeit in public spaces) for behavior that might compromise the company's image and productivity. We might imagine that sharing health data could present the tempting possibility of manipulating the workforce for increased profits.

Section Eight: The Rebellion

"This blog has empowered me to flush my remaining pills down the toilet. The insidious, cumulative, and destructive effects of the so-called new generation of birth control pills are terrifying on a woman's emotional state. I'm calling them "Stepford Pills." It is so eerie to read of other's nearly identical reactions." – Jane

The number of pill refugees is growing but this group continues to be dismissed as ungrateful hypochondriacs. The tales with the most drama are more often published and glean the biggest audience and this can have the adverse effect of causing women to think that if they are not experiencing side effects as frightening or intense as those described that they must not be experiencing any kind of negative impact. If we don't have a blood clot, we think we must be okay.

Women are forging paths independently to find alternatives for pregnancy prevention and treating menstrual health problems outside of the medical establishment. They are pioneers but so often isolated, concerned that they will be viewed as irresponsible, prudish or misguided. In the US, to take this path with no religious reasoning is to accept a position requiring constant self-justification.

Those looking to deny access to contraception to women and roll back abortion rights were defeated in the 2012 US election. When President Obama won a second term a cheer went up that expressed the feeling that women could keep dominion over their own bodies. They could still choose. But what are their choices? They are choices presented to them by rich, old, white men and women, chosen for us by rich, old, white men going back centuries through history.

Gray argues that men and women live within cycles that have no connection to the structure of our society. Men are tuned most deeply into the solar cycle across the seasons and will feel, think and work differently from summer to winter. They are also synched in to the monthly tidal pull within their own bodies and through the women with whom they connect. A man's pre-ovulation phase is spring; ovulation during the summer and their menstrual phase is in the winter. Women are also affected by the solar cycle and their reaction to monthly changes will depend on the time of year.

Gray encourages her clients to work on synchronizing their cycle to the lunar phases by becoming aware of the changes and preparing their body to meld with the appearance of the new moon and the full moon. Women have success using techniques like sleeping with a light on (called "night lighting") and sleeping in a pitch-dark room at appropriate periods of the month. In modern society we so rarely live in the complete darkness of a new or so-called "dark moon" that we must create it. The practice is based on the theory that women living in a past or present pre-industrial society would frequently ovulate with the full moon and menstruate with the new moon. This belief assumes women would sleep exposed to the moon's light rather than in a windowless cave or shelter or in a windowed shelter with no way to block light.

Aside from artificial light, there are many factors that can prevent women from experiencing regular cycles. Endocrine disrupting chemicals in food, shampoo, and furniture and, of course, the cycle damage done by hormonal contraception also takes a toll. It is possible that without these interruptions women would generally synch with the moon phases.

Gray believes that women with a similar sense of purpose and those that have a similar outlook and approach to life are more likely to synchronize. Their emotional connection and shared ideals have an effect on whether this will occur. Although the only contemporary research available emphasizes physical proximity as provoking synchronization, it seems it might not be as simple as an equation of proximity, schedule or pheromones.

The culture of shame, disgust and indifference to the menstrual cycle has its own impact on women's experience, physically and emotionally, of their cycles. The "bio-feedback" loop produces stress that then causes health issues to arise or worsen, thus making a woman's cycle more difficult. The hate or fear we are taught to feel about our menstruation is insidious. Gray considers, "There is no basis in modern culture for being a constantly changing and transitioning person. Consistency is valued above all."

Psychologist Joan Chrisler writes that sameness has been sanctified as a standard although this goes against human nature. "Change, not constancy, should be seen as normal," she argues.

Anthropologist Chris Knight believes that Gray offers a positive opportunity for women but her teachings present only half an answer to the question of women's suppression in society through science. In *Blood Relations: Menstruation and The Origins of Culture* Knight explores the possibility that in ancient cultures women synchronized their cycles and in so doing created the foundations of civilization. Our justification for the inevitability or naturalness of capitalism, he theorizes, is a construct based in Darwinism.

As a Marxist, he proposes we reassess the origins of our culture and consider that change and upheaval, specifically overturning the system of how we live now, might be more inevitable and natural than acceptance of the status quo. Women established our collective and collaborative humanity, he argues, by creating a revolution based on a sex-strike. He theorizes that women struck a collaborative bargain that held the community together: if men did not bring meat back from the hunt, they did not have sex.

During the new moon women lived amongst their mothers, sisters, children and fellow women whilst the men took to the hunt to bring back food for all. They might have withdrawn to a menstrual hut, living in very close quarters. When they returned, at the full moon, women who were not pregnant, breast-feeding or older were ovulating and ready to have procreative sex.

How, Knight asks, did women get the men to do this work for them? The sex-strike was produced through synchronized menstruation. The women's period blood would signal to the men "no sex" but their scheme would only work if all women produced blood at the same time. The sense of duty to others in a community, and as such civilization, was established this way.

Of his feminist perspective Knight explains, "Influenced by friends and comrades who were feminists, I naturally felt feminism of any variety to be a liberating political force. But for the women I was closest to the construction of "female males" was not what the struggle was all about, any more than joining the capitalists was the essence of working-class emancipation. The struggle was more about refusing to collaborate with the whole masculinist political set-up, organizing autonomously as women, drawing on support for real change from the wider class struggle - and fighting to bring men as allies into a world transformed on women's terms."

Knight understands the popularity of menstrual suppression through hormonal contraceptives as indicative of society's requirement that women "suppress and deny their own biology as a condition of feeling liberated." The drugs and devices are part of a history that required women be isolated from each other in order to be ruled over by men, "Like workers denied collective control over their own labor, mothers were prevented from synchronizing their cycles or menstrual flows and prevented from benefitting collectively from the potency of their bodily processes."

The fault line running through mainstream feminism is that feminists have made the choice to encourage women to make their way in this society, and be "like men" in order to assimilate and belong.

Capitalism is built on a clock that regards time in terms of money. This understanding of time is not based on the original, essential clock of the moon phases. Modern society, as Swift also argued, is always on "full moon time," demanding consistent productivity. Knight believes women to be more connected to the original clock than men because of their biology.

Although he argues that women make the choice to use the pill from a justified viewpoint – one that reveals that they feel they can only be comfortable and accepted if they suppress their cycle – he likens the acceptance of menstrual suppression drugs to the situation of black South Africans during Apartheid. At that time it was seen that some would try to argue they were "not *that* black" in order to fit into the oppressive system. Women are expected to be "as good as men" and live up to that impossible ideal.

Schlain proposes an interconnected theory, that menstruation taught humanity the concept of time. He also theorizes that groups of women synchronizing their menstrual cycles allowed them to assert female equality.

Schlain also believes that for much of our history women were able to connect their cycles to the lunar month. He suggests that most women had cycles of this length and would ovulate on the full moon and menstruate at the new moon. In agreement with Knight he suggests women harnessed power over sex through synchronization. They used the combined power of saying "No." Shlain goes as far as to say that the angry reaction of men to women's self-control when it comes to sex in the face of their own lack of self-control is the root of misogyny.

From a growing understanding of the pattern of menstruation came the concept of time and with it the understanding of mortality as well as the connected desire to produce children that might secure a sort of immortality. Schlain writes, "The institution of patriarchy came into existence because men needed, first, to control women's sexuality and, second, to control women's reproductive rights. A man's control over the former ensured that he could relieve his intolerable itch on terms favorable to his sex; control of the second assured his place in posterity."

Knight theorizes that men stole the ritual of menstruation from women by reenacting it themselves. Australian Aboriginal men believe women do not experience a "real" period and demand that they are isolated from each other during menstruation. The men through self-mutilation reenact period bleeding together in synchronization as their own ritual separate to the women. Knight suggests men overthrew the order that was established by women and instigated a system of male domination in its place by co-opting this element of women's power.

It is a theory that has echoes in the development of a "fake period" for women using the pill, which acts as a substitute for their cycle. Instead of celebratory rituals around menstruation, women now have the ritual, established for them by men, of taking a pill every day.

"Women were being made to fear their blood potency. Their own reproductive powers were being alienated from them, taken from them, turned into their opposite and constructed as a force to oppose all women," writes Knight. In modern society we have done away with kinship or communal relationships and the understanding of collective experience partly because menstruation represents kinship so essentially.

What would a society "transformed on women's terms" look like? A culture that is habitable for female biology and does not require women to medicate to assimilate. What if women did not adapt to the system but decided to change it, starting with tuning back into their bodies and their collective power?

Knight believes in "the inevitable potential for women to connect up and present a massive force if they were all tapped into their cycles." Coming off hormonal contraceptives could provide the catalyst to change that system from the strength of collective experience.

In Martin's essay titled 'Premenstrual Syndrome: Discipline, Anger and Work in Late Industrial Societies' she explores the potential for PMS to be seen as a positive force to incite rebellion. If women are less tolerant pre-menstrual of their duties and discipline and more in touch with their bodies there is the potential for that intolerance to be channeled into collective change.

Martin writes of the social and scientific translation of PMS, "It is the women who malfunction and must have their hormone imbalances fixed, not the organization of society and work that might be transformed so that it could demand less constant discipline and productivity."

Hormonal contraceptives are supposed to level women, and for some they are leveled so as to feel depressed, for others the suppression produces, along with panic attacks and fear, bouts of intense rage. The drugs disseminate the rage through the month; mix it with depression, fear and self-doubt, making it unworkable and rootless.

Martin writes that menstruation is the "moment of truth which will not sustain lies." Martin describes how in the days before her period she is hyper-aware that "she is discriminated against as a woman." She realizes that her partner, her children and society at large put inhuman demands on her in all areas of life. She cannot go on this way, Martin decides, things must change: "If these kinds of causes are the root of the unnamed anger that seems to afflict women, and if they could be named and known, maybe a cleaner, more productive anger would seem to arise from within women, tying them together as a common oppressed instead of sending them individually to the doctor as patients to be fixed."

The emotional turmoil women experience as a result of hormonal birth control should bond and connect them, providing an opportunity for women to understand themselves as collectively mistreated by a system working against their needs. The anger women feel when they discover their contraception has caused them suffering can be directed outward and shared.

In a sense these drugs have produced a fake PMS akin to the fake period that separates us from experiencing our body's changes. Women report feeling anger and directing this at their partners, friends, anyone they otherwise love and trust. The feeling borne of suppression is detached from its root and this causes women to question their views. Even after coming off the pill women might be afraid of any PMS-like anger they feel because of their trauma and be anxious to not examine these feelings when they arise and instead dismiss them.

Martin argues that society copes with a rise of anger in women by "insisting that the rage and rebellion, as well as the physical pain, will all be cured by the administration of drugs." Women's desire to go on strike from their duties, over-burdened as they so often are with paid work, housework, and childcare, is called "maladaptive discontent." We can be made to adapt through medication.

To those who see the time positively, menstruation presents an opportunity to connect to inner sources of creativity, intuition and self-knowledge. Fertility awareness teacher Talibah Ndidi tutors women in the importance of withdrawing from family, friends and working life during menstruation in order to be able to tap into these abilities as they are amplified. It is a time, she claims, for women to look inward and seek their purpose. If they are prevented from doing so then they will react to the repression negatively. In order to gain seclusion in her own life Ndidi wears a red bracelet during her period to let her friends and family know.

Capitalism does not support a monthly time of low productivity as defined within strict parameters of profit making. Self-knowledge connected to the body and the collective experience is viewed as a threat. Ndidi believes women can take advantage of menstrual synchronization to experience a very physical, visceral connection with each other.

This proposition, of course, is not inclusive of those women who are not menstruating due to their stage in life whether that be pre-pubescence, pregnancy or menopause. This is why an emphasis on body literacy above and beyond cycle charting is important. All phases of the female life have the undercurrent of change. The female body changes from girl to woman and in order to form another life and through the end of menstruation. Change is fundamental to the female experience.

The Los Angeles based all-female bicycle brigade, the Ovarian Psycos, is made up of young women of color determined to create a safe space to address problems in their communities. During their monthly Luna Rides the group members, along with other women outside of the group including those who self-identify as women, ride together through the city under a full moon. They end the events with a "talking circle" at which they share information about that month's cause, be that incidents of violence against women in their neighborhood or sexual health issues. The meeting mimics traditional moon ceremonies with the use of sage for cleansing and bonding rituals.

The name of the collective, created by founder Xela, is a deliberate repurposing of the oppressive medical interpretations of the reproductive cycle. The women wear bandannas over their faces painted with illustrations of a womb and ovaries. With the motto "Ovaries so big we don't need balls" they invented the "Ovarian Gang Sign" for which they make a sign of the ovaries and womb with their hands held in front of their bodies. The sign is an act of reclamation and subversion of gang culture for positive and purposeful ends. Their mission reads, "We envision a world where women of color are change agents who create and maintain holistic health within themselves and in their respective communities for present and future generations."

Each new cycle presents the opportunity for change. Women share that they find it is easier to consciously let go of unhelpful and stale feelings, thoughts and ideas at the transition into a new cycle. The introversion of menstruation can bring in an awareness of the world as a whole. There might be a rush of empathy for others and a heightened consciousness of suffering and oppression. This is Martin's "moment of truth."

Menstrual "outing" is a recent evolution of the menstrual activism movement. To admit publicly "I am menstruating today" is a radical action in our culture. Enthusiasts of this brand of activism encourage women to announce it through their Facebook status, or by wearing a badge or tee shirt.

Student Stephanie Robinson writes, "I outed myself in a women's studies class, stating that I was menstruating, and the reaction that I got from the students in an upper division women's studies sexuality class was very surprising. Many women looked embarrassed for me, some scoffed and others just ignored my statement, which made me think, if in this supposedly forward thinking space, how are we still getting these reactions to menstruation?"

Swift and her partner teach couples that are concerned about the side effects of hormonal contraceptives how to transition to fertility awareness. Both the man and the woman of the couple are taught how to use diet, exercise and herbalism to make the change. They are also both told how to track the woman's cycle and know how to note the fertile time.

Through this Swift finds that both men and women become conscious of the pressure put on them to be consistently "on" and ready for both sex and work. The couple might see how they both feel the expectation to have a lot of sex rather than the sex they want. Our society conditions us to value quantity over quality in this area of life as in all others.

Comparatively at work they will be aware their boss values

the early start and staying late, the amount of time spent at the desk, over the quality of the work output.

Swift sees that coming off hormonal contraceptives signals to people that they will have less sex, although the truth varies. However accepting and considering this often makes people feel uncomfortable. Women and men may feel they reclaim the right to have sex when they want to and not when they feel they ought to and to not use sex as an easy and acceptable substitute for conversation or another form of connection. The promise of hormonal contraceptives to provide the freedom of no-strings sex is internalized.

Studies into the impact of hormonal birth control on libido often focuses on frequency as a marker and that frequency tends to go up when a woman starts on a drug or device. If we take a pill every day to prevent pregnancy but only have sex once a month it can throw that action into the stark relief and make it questionable.

The pressure on women to take hormonal contraceptives is not only in the insidious pro-pill culture. Women report to Swift being openly threatened and strong-armed into choosing hormonal methods. They endure harassment at Planned Parenthood clinics and blackmail by doctors. Women say they have had to make multiple appointments to persuade their practitioner to remove a device or provide an alternative like a diaphragm.

One woman, Swift describes, desperately wanted her Mirena removed after suffering serious emotional issues but her doctor responded that he would only perform the procedure if she agreed to be sterilized. She felt so weighed down by the depression and anxiety she did not have the strength to question him. She was coerced into sterilization.

Couples learning fertility awareness extend their teaching to the day-to-day practice of the method. Swift encourages the man to take his partner's temperature every morning and chart this information. The woman is responsible for marking the cervical mucus changes and adding other information that is relevant.

This makes the method even more effective at preventing pregnancy as it brings the male partner in on the knowledge. He is aware of when his partner is fertile and supports the avoidance penetrative sex or use of barrier methods. As a system, it promotes trust and openness. It also eliminates the sense of the burden sitting solely on the shoulders of the woman to be responsible for preventing a pregnancy.

"Through history we've always blamed women for getting pregnant even though it's men that are fertile every single day. This cooperation liberates women from that, but it also liberates men in letting them know that they too can decide to be unavailable. They can have less sex and be just as masculine, despite what they've been taught. We don't just need women's liberation, we need a people's liberation," says Swift.

We need to democratize the knowledge of fertility awareness. We must get to a point at which teen girls don't think their cervical mucus must be a sign of infection. The New York state pilot program to allow high school teens access to the morning-after emergency contraceptive without parental consent is pioneering but this development along with access to abortion services needs to be supported by a culture of body literacy and truly informed choice, otherwise it may only lead to more teens being put on LARCs. The more education there is, the less need for emergency contraceptives and abortion services. However, these options must be there for women's agency. An emergency pill taken once or twice a year is better than a birth control pill taken every day.

The self-proclaimed leader in hormonal contraceptives, Bayer, is also the world's leading agrochemical company and the seventh biggest seed production company. Its nicotine-based pesticides, neo-nicotinoids, are linked to the demise of the bee population threatening the future of agriculture and the natural eco-system. In Germany, Italy and France suspensions of use of these pesticides have been voiced, but the research is not acknowledged in the UK or US. The findings are refuted by the manufacturers with claims that if used "correctly" there is no impact on the bees. As with the research behind blood clot risk and drospirenone-containing drugs the government bodies have gone with Bayer's own proposed research, rather than that presented to them by independent researchers.

Eco-feminism argues that the insistence of dominion over women is connected inextricably to Western patriarchal capitalist culture's oppression of the natural environment. Eco-feminism demands that a co-existing environmentalism is essential for women's liberation. This assertion is founded in the history of oppressed races and classes, not only women, being associated with concepts of "Nature." Their oppression is histor-ically justified by this connection.

Eco-feminists believe that until we accept and nurture our human link to nature, especially the strong connection of women through the lunar cycle, we cannot prevent and overthrow the dominion over women. Working with, instead of against nature, is the future for humanity and resistance to this will only lead to destruction. It is argued that as nature is approached like a machine, women and men are manipulated as though they too are machines, all in the pursuit of capitalist progress.

Amy Sedgwick, founder of the eco-feminist collective Red Tent Sisters, developed the 'Green Your Birth Control in 30 Days' online seminar series that embodies the democratization of fertility awareness and body literacy. In an article titled 'Coming Off the Pill: The Final Frontier for Women Pursuing Holistic Health' she speaks to those women who eat organic, avoid chemical-laden products and see themselves as eco-conscious, "Aside from "the pill is making me crazy" the most common reason I hear from women choosing to switch to natural birth control is that the pill no longer fits with their values."

Subverting Faulkner's assertion that "women are tied to the earth" Sedgwick suggests women "live closer to the Earth, live in synch with the Earth and live in respect of the Earth" for the good of their health, fertility and for the good of the environment.

Gandhi prayed every day, "Make me more womanly – make me more feminine." We can speculate he was drawing on the eco-feminist idea that women carry a culture of caring and sharing, from nature or from nurture, and that is subsumed in modern society. Both men and women could embrace these elements of humanness and deny the dichotomy of male and female, nature and culture. Eco-feminists believe, as Knight does, that there was a time when cooperation and not competition were vital to the human experience and that it is possible for us to tap back into those origins.

In this post-recession era we have seen institutions questioned and criticized in the mainstream arena. The system broke and its innards were exposed.

The food industry for one is under fire with the meat and dairy lobbies in the spotlight for their domination over our diets. Documentaries like *Forks Over Knives* and *Food Inc.* reached massive audiences of people eager to be healthy and environ-mentally kind. The focus is on what we put in our bodies.

The pill makes women feel disconnected, repressed and deadened. Through reconnecting with our bodies we are in a better position to connect with others, and with the world. As you will have seen through these pages, coming off the pill is an "awakening" for many women. Hormonal birth control can create a sense of indifference and detachment. If we suffer with panic attacks, agoraphobia and anxiety we direct our energy and emotions into this black hole. It is a hard place to return from with confidence when the culture does not admit to the validity of your experience.

Taking the pill seemed to me, for a long time, like the easy way out despite the consequences to my mental and physical health.

If I started taking it again I would be back in control, I could regain the bigger breasts, flatter stomach, clearer skin and glossier hair that Yaz had given me. I would be acceptable regardless of my anxiety or my rage, as long as I looked good and right.

Bartky writes in her essay 'Modernization of Patriarchical Power,' "To have a body felt to be feminine – a body socially constructed through the appropriate practices - is in most cases crucial to a woman's sense of herself as female and her sense of herself as an existing individual." Rejecting the pill threw me into a space in which I did not know who I could be. As I wrote in those first weeks of blogging – who am I when I'm not on the pill? Ridding myself of the pill made me ask a lot more questions than just this.

A motto of the Berkeley Women's Health Collective was "Our Strength is in Our Health." The choice to come off the pill and be well rather than sick does not have to be a political action. To politicize this suggests that achieving personal wellness is not a good enough end in itself.

Achieving wellness is not only a means to an end of protest, resistance or social change, it is important in its own right. That wellness does not have to made useful or productive. Women should not feel they have to affiliate with any way of thinking to make the transition.

When I came off the pill it was to feel better first and foremost, and that is reason enough. I did, however, decide to share the experience in the hope other women might learn from my transition. It is only through wellness that we have the strength of mind and body to take action in our own lives and collectively.

In a sense, rejecting hormonal contraceptives is, in our culture, a necessarily political act, but it is up to us to decide what we create from that point. The feelings of anger and awareness that we feel can be used to benefit other women.

A phrase was created as part of the work of the Occupy movement – Occupy Yourself.

To some this means acting as a vigilant and engaged citizen. For others it requires critically analyzing the thoughts and beliefs you have long held to be true. I had to examine my long held beliefs about my body, my femininity and my cycle to be able to get off and stay off the pill.

That oft repeated phrase "Be the change you want to see in the world" grew to have a very specific meaning for me. On the pill I was stagnant - physically, mentally and emotionally. I would get stuck in both feelings and thoughts. I could not think clearly. I could not progress. Off the pill, my body is going through changes throughout the month. I experience the waves and peaks, the ebbs and flows and all of this moves me. This movement is energizing and galvanizing.

I feel in this way that I am truly occupying myself. Every new cycle spurs action in me. I encourage you to step out of the system and back into yourself. It could be a revolution from the inside out.

List of references and additional reading

Pope, Alexandra and Bennet, Jane, *The Pill: Are You Sure It's For You?* Allen and Unwin, 2009

Seaman, Barbara, *The Doctor's Case Against the Pill*, PH Wyden, 1969

Project on Government Oversight
http://pogo.org/

Pharmalot articles on Bayer law suits by Ed Silverman
http://www.pharmalot.com

Ehrenreich, Barbara and English, Dierdre, *For Her Own Good: Two Centuries of Experts Advice For Women*, Anchor Books, 2005

Seaman, Barbara, *The Greatest Experiment Ever Performed on Women: Exploding the Estrogen Myth*, Hyperion, 2003

Dalton, Katherine, *Once A Month: Understanding and Treating PMS*, Fontana Paperbacks 1978

Houppert, Karen, T*he Curse: Confronting the Last Unmentionable Taboo: Menstruation*, Farrar, Staus and Giroux, 1999

Bobel, Chris, *New Blood: Third Wave Feminism and the Politics of Menstruation*, Rutgers University Press, 2010

Martin, Emily, *The Woman in the Body: A Cultural Analysis of Reproduction*, Beacon Press, 1987

Wolf, Naomi, *The Beauty Myth: How Images of Beauty Are Used Against Women*, Perennial, 2002

Justisse Healthworks for Women
http://www.justisse.ca/

Lalonde, Megan and Matus, Geraldine, *Coming off the Pill, the Patch, the Shot and Other Hormonal Contraceptives*, Justisse Healthworks for Women, 2007

Matus, Geraldine, *Justisse Method: Fertility Awareness and Body Literacy: A User's Guide*, Justisse Healthworks for Women, 2009

Weshler, Toni, *Taking Charge of Your Fertility: A Guide To Charting*

Your Fertility Signals, Quill, 2002

Singer, Katie, *The Garden of Fertility*, Avery, 2004

Vliet, Elizabeth Lee, *It's My Ovaries, Stupid!*, Evans and Company, 2003

Eldridge, Laura, *In Our Control: A Complete Guide To Contraceptive Choices for Women*, Seven Stories Press, 2010

Faludi, Susan, *Backlash: The Undeclared War Against American Women*, Three Rivers Press, 1991

Oudshoorn, Nelly, *Beyond the Natural Body: An Archeology of Sex Hormones*, Routledge, 1994

Society for Menstrual Cycle Research blog: re:Cycling
http://menstruationresearch.org/blog

Coutinho, Elsimar and Segal, Sheldon, *Is Menstruation Obsolete?*, Oxford University Press, 1999

Kissling, Elizabeth, *Capitalizing on the Curse: The Business of Menstruation*, Lynne Rienner Publishers, 2006

Kissling, Elizabeth, What Does Not Kill You Makes You Stronger: Young Women's Online Conversations about Quitting the Pill in Meredith Nash, *Reframing Reproduction*, Palgrave Macmillan, 2014 (in press)

Bitch guest blog: Reproductive Writes series
http://bitchmagazine.org/profile/holly-grigg-spall

Center for Menstrual Cycle and Ovulation Research
http://www.cemcor.ubc.ca/

Prior, Jerilynn and Baxter, Susan, *The Estrogen Errors: Why Progesterone is Better for Women's Health*, Praeger Publishers, 2009

Rako, Susan, *No More Periods?: The Risks of Menstrual Suppression*, Harmony Books, 2003

The Business of Being Born, documentary, Abby Epstein and Ricki Lake

Hartmann, Betsy, *Reproductive Rights and Wrongs: The Global Politics of Population Control*, Perennial Library, 1987

Tyler May, Elaine, *America and The Pill: A History of Promise, Peril and Liberation*, Basic Books, 2010

Walter, Natasha, *Living Dolls: The Return of Sexism*, Virago, 2010

Levy, Ariel, *Female Chauvinist Pigs: Women and the Rise of Raunch Culture*, Free Press, 2005

Gray, Miranda, *The Optimized Woman: Using Your Menstrual Cycle to Achieve Success and Fulfillment*, O-Books, 2009

Orgasm Inc, documentary, Liz Canner

Foucault, Michel, *Discipline and Punish: The Birth of The Prison*, Vintage Books, 1995

Ehrenreich, Barbara and English, Deirdre, *Complaints and Disorders: The Sexual Politics of Sickness*, The Feminist Press, 1973

Tiefer, Leonore, *Sex is Not a Natural Act and Other Essays*, Westview Press, 1995

Tiefer, Leonore and Kaschak, Ellyn, *A New View Of Women's Sexual Problems*, The Haworth Press, 2001

Ehrenreich, Barbara and Hess, Elizabeth and Jacobs, Gloria, *Re-Making Love: The Feminization of Sex*, Anchor Books, 1986

Norgren, Tiana, *Abortion Before Birth Control: The Politics of Reproduction in Japan*, Princeton University Press, 2001

Takeshita, Chikako, *The Global Biopolitics of the IUD: How Science Constructs Contraceptive Users and Women's Bodies*, MIT Press, 2012

Downer, Carol and Chalker, Rebecca, *A Woman's Book of Choices*, Four Walls Eight Windows, 1992

Downer, Carol, *A New View of a Woman's Body from The Federation of Feminist Women's Health Centers*, Feminist Health Press, 1991

Buckley, Thomas and Gottlieb, Alma, *Blood Magic: The Anthropology of Menstruation*, University of California Press, 1988

The Moon Inside You, documentary, Diana Fabianova

Period. The End of Menstruation, documentary, Giovanna Chesler

Knight, Chris, *Blood Relations: Menstruation and the Origins of Culture*, Yale University Press, 1991

Bennett, Jane and Naish, Francesca, The Natural Fertility Management Contraception Kit

Gauthier, Isabelle and Vinebaum, Lisa, *Hot Pantz: DIY Gynecology*, Blood Sisters Reproduction

Nickerson, Brittany Wood, *Sacred and Mysterious: Healing Wisdom and Herbal Lore for Those Who Menstruate*, Everyday Living Series, 2012

Swift, Katja, Plant Healer magazine series
http://commonwealthherbs.com/pharmacy/homework/the-lunareturn-series-from-plant-healer-magazine/

Tone, Andrea, *Devices and Desires: A History of Contraceptives in America*, Hill and Wang, 2001

Bartky, Sandra Lee, *Femininity and Domination: Studies in the Phenomenology of Oppression*, Routledge, 1990

Sawicki, Jana, *Disciplining Foucault: Feminism, Power, and The Body*, Routledge, 1991

Schlain, Leonard, *Sex, Time, and Power: How Women's Sexuality Shaped Human Evolution*, Penguin, 2003

Ussher, Jane, *Managing the Monstrous Feminine: Regulating the Reproductive Body*, Routledge, 2007

Red Tent Sisters
http://redtentsisters.com/

The Shodhini Institute
http://shodhini.blogspot.com/

Women's Health Specialists – Feminist Women's Health Centers of California
http://www.womenshealthspecialists.org/

Fertility Awareness Center of New York
http://www.fertaware.com/

Ovarian Psycos
http://ovarianpsycos.com/

'Coming off the pill: a guide' at the Sweetening the Pill blog http://sweeteningthepill.blogspot.com/2012/03/could-furor-over-contraception-spark.html

Contemporary culture has eliminated both the concept of the public and the figure of the intellectual. Former public spaces – both physical and cultural – are now either derelict or colonized by advertising. A cretinous anti-intellectualism presides, cheerled by expensively educated hacks in the pay of multinational corporations who reassure their bored readers that there is no need to rouse themselves from their interpassive stupor. The informal censorship internalized and propagated by the cultural workers of late capitalism generates a banal conformity that the propaganda chiefs of Stalinism could only ever have dreamt of imposing. Zer0 Books knows that another kind of discourse – intellectual without being academic, popular without being populist – is not only possible: it is already flourishing, in the regions beyond the striplit malls of so-called mass media and the neurotically bureaucratic halls of the academy. Zer0 is committed to the idea of publishing as a making public of the intellectual. It is convinced that in the unthinking, blandly consensual culture in which we live, critical and engaged theoretical reflection is more important than ever before.